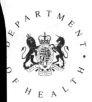

The Prevention of Depression and Anxiety

The role of the primary care team

A conference organised by the Prevention Project at MIND and the Department of Health and chaired by the Royal College of General Practitioners

Edited by Rachel Jenkins, Jennifer Newton and Robyn Young

London: HMSO

© Crown copyright 1992
Applications for reproduction should be made to HMSO
First published 1992

ISBN 0 11 321450 2

Preface

This conference, on Prevention of Depression and Anxiety – the Role of the Primary Care Team, is the second in a series sponsored by the Department of Health on mental illness and the primary care services, as was reported in the 'Caring for People' White Paper[1]. The series is being published, and aims to identify ways of improving prevention, detection and management by the primary care team.

The first conference in the series, on Counselling in General Practice, was held in collaboration with the Institute of Psychiatry and the Royal College of General Practitioners in May 1989[2]; the third, on the Primary Care of Schizophrenia, was held in collaboration with Research and Development for Psychiatry, and the Royal College of General Practitioners in June 1990[3].

This conference, on Prevention of Depression and Anxiety – the Role of the Primary Care Team, was held in collaboration with the Prevention Project at MIND and the Royal College of General Practitioners in March 1990, in order to bring together expert knowledge in the field and stimulate developments in primary care. We hope that this publication will be helpful to primary care practitioners at a time when the primary care of mental illness is in a very exciting phase of development.

RACHEL JENKINS, JENNIFER NEWTON AND ROBYN YOUNG

[1] Department of Health 1989
    Caring for People
    Community Care in the Next Decade and Beyond
    LONDON: HMSO

[2] R Corney and R Jenkins 1992
    Counselling in General Practice
    Routledge (In Press)

[3] R Jenkins, V Field, R Young 1992
    Primary Care of Schizophrenia
    LONDON: HMSO

Chapter List

	Page
Preface	iii
Foreword A Dr John Reed	xiii
Foreword B Dr Colin Waine	xvi

Chapter 1   1
Depression and Anxiety in Primary Care: The Epidemiological Evidence
(*Professor Anthony Mann*)

Chapter 2   11
Depression and Anxiety: An Overview of Preventive Strategies
(*Dr Rachel Jenkins*)

Chapter 3   22
Life Events and Social Support: Possibilities for Primary Prevention
(*Professor George Brown*)

Chapter 4   33
Early Diagnosis and Secondary Prevention
(*Professor David Goldberg*)

Chapter 5   39
Teaching Psychiatric Interview Skills to General Practitioners
(*Dr Linda Gask*)

Chapter 6   46
The Computer will see you now: Meeting the Challenge of Hidden Psychiatric Morbidity in General Practice
(*Dr Alastair Wright*)

Chapter 7   57
Implications for General Practice Training and Education
(*Professor Paul Freeling*)

Chapter 8   68
Crisis Support: Utilising Resources
(*Dr Jennifer Newton*)

	Page
Chapter 9A Counselling in General Practice: Options for Action A. Clinical Psychology *(Meredith Robson)*	77
Chapter 9B Counselling in General Practice: Options for Action B. A Social Worker's Point of View *(Mary Burke)*	82
Chapter 9C Counselling in General Practice: Options for Action C. Person-Centred Counselling *(Christine Manzi)*	87
Chapter 9D Counselling in General Practice: Options for Action D. The Nurse Practitioner/Counsellor *(Nicola McFarland)*	91
Chapter 10A Liaison in Primary Care: Early Detection of Difficulties A. Preventing Child Neglect *(Dr Keith Beswick and Mrs Pauline Richardson)*	95
Chapter 10B Liaison Between Providers of Primary Care: Early Detection of Difficulties B. Predicting Postnatal Depression *(Dr Deborah Sharp)*	101
Chapter 11A Liaison between Primary and Secondary Care Teams Towards Early Intervention *(Dr Geraldine Strathdee)*	113
Chapter 11B Liaison between Primary and Secondary Care Teams Towards Early Intervention B. Assertive Help for Inner City Distress *(Steve Onyett)*	124
Chapter 12A Health Information A. A Health Education Library in General Practice *(Clare Pace)*	131
Chapter 12B Health Information B. Self-Help Health Information Services *(Robert Gann)*	135

	Page
Chapter 13A Linking with Voluntary and Community Resources A. Home-Start Consultancy *(Mrs Margaret Harrison)*	140
Chapter 13B Linking with Voluntary and Community Resources B. Camden Tranquilliser Services *(Ruby Tovet)*	145
Chapter 13C Linking with Voluntary and Community Resources C. A GP's Perspective *(Dr Katy Gardner)*	150
Chapter 14 Mental Health Promotion in General Practice *(Dr Caryle Steen)*	155

Contributors List

Dr John Reed
Senior Principal Medical Officer
Health Care (Medical)
Department of Health
Wellington House
133–155 Waterloo Road
LONDON
SE1 8UG

Dr Colin Waine, OBE, FRCGP
Chairman of Council
Royal College of General Practitioners
14 Princes Gate
Hyde Park
LONDON
SW7 1PU

Professor Anthony Mann
Professor of Epidemiological Psychiatry
Institute of Psychiatry
De Crespigny Park
Denmark Hill
LONDON
SE5 8AF

Dr Rachel Jenkins
Principal Medical Officer
Health Care (Medical)
Department of Health
Wellington House
133–155 Waterloo Road
LONDON
SE1 8UG

Professor George Brown
Department of Social Policy and Social Science
Royal Holloway and Bedford New College
11 Bedford Square
LONDON
WC1B 3RA

Professor David Goldberg
Professor of Psychiatry
University of Manchester
Department of Psychiatry
Withington Hospital
West Didsbury
MANCHESTER
M20 8LR

Dr Linda Gask
Senior Lecturer in Psychiatry
Avondale Unit
Royal Preston Hospital
PO Box 66
Sharoe Green Lane
Preston
PR2 4HT

Dr Alastair Wright
Royal College of General Practitioners
14 Princes Gate
Hyde Park
LONDON
SW7 1PU

Professor Paul Freeling
Division of General Practice and Primary Care
St George's Hospital Medical School
University of London
Cranmer Terrace
LONDON
SW17 0RE

Dr Jennifer Newton
Primary Health Care Project Officer
Health Education Authority
Hamilton House
Mabledon Place
LONDON
WC1H 9TX

Meredith Robson
Department of Psychology
Charing Cross Hospital
Fulham Palace Road
LONDON W6

Mary Burke
The Surgery
241 Westbourne Grove
LONDON W11 2SE

Christine Manzi
Theobold Centre
121 Theobold Street
Boreham Wood
HERTS
WD6 4PU

Nicola MacFarland
The Medical Centre
2 Garway Road
LONDON
W2 4NH

Dr Keith Beswick and Mrs Pauline Richardson
Didcot Health Centre
Asbury Medical Centre
Britwell Road
DIDCOT
Oxfordshire
OX11 7JH

Dr Deborah Sharp
Department of General Practice
United and Dental Schools of Guys and St Thomas's Hospitals
80 Kennington Road
LONDON
SE11 6SP

Dr Geraldine Strathdee
Consultant Psychiatrist
Maudsley Hospital
Denmark Hill
LONDON
SE5 8AF

Steve Onyett
Teamwork Project Manager
Research and Development for Psychiatry
134–138 Borough High Street
LONDON SE1 1LB

Clare Pace
Dib Lane Surgery
112A Dib Lane
LEEDS
LS8 3AY

Robert Gann
Director
The Help for Health Trust
Highcroft Cottage
Romsey Road
WINCHESTER
SO22 5DH

Margaret Harrison
Director
HOME-START Consultancy
2 Salisbury Road
LEICESTER
LE1 7QR

Ruby Tovet
Camden Tranquilliser Services
Barnes House
9–15 Camden Road
LONDON
NW1 9LQ

Dr Katy Gardner
Princes Park Health Centre
Bentley Road
LIVERPOOL
L8 3TX

Dr Caryle Steen
The James Wigg Practice
Kentish Town Health Centre
2 Bartholomew Road
LONDON
NW5 2AJ

Foreword A

JOHN REED, Senior Principal Medical Officer, Department of Health, London

As part of the Government's response to the Griffiths Report White Paper, *Caring for People*[1], Ministers indicated that they would examine primary health care to see what practical steps could be taken to improve it. The Department of Health/MIND/RCGP conference on the *Prevention of Anxiety and Depression* was arranged as part of that examination. The response to the conference – the breadth of which is reflected in the chapters of this book – showed widespread agreement among the many professions and organisations involved, that primary mental health care is of central importance to the future of mental health services.

The reasons for this are by now fairly well known. GPs come into contact with, and are responsible for treating the bulk of psychiatric disorder in the population, and only a small proportion of the mentally disordered who consult GPs reach the specialist psychiatric services. Patients consulting their general practitioners with psychiatric disorder outnumber consultant outpatient attenders by 10:1, and psychiatric admissions by 100:1. Demonstrable psychosocial difficulties are present in 1 in 3 of all GP attenders, and the annual prevalence of depression and anxiety in the adult population is very high (between 15 and 25 per cent depending on the clinical criteria adopted).

Furthermore, the primary care setting provides the greatest opportunities for both primary and secondary prevention of mental illness. It is at the primary care level that recognition of patient risk factors and detection of illness usually occurs. Primary preventive strategies include identification and support of those at high risk of depression eg the elderly, bereaved, socially isolated, physically disabled, the blind and the deaf. Secondary preventive strategies include the prompt treatment of those who are depressed and anxious. Depression, which is frequently unrecognised and untreated, has a better prognosis if it is identified by the GP. It is therefore crucial to improve detection and management in order to avoid the consequences of untreated depression, eg an increased risk of suicide and parasuicide, marital breakdown, and considerable occupational problems such as sickness absence, labour turnover, problems with colleagues, poor performance and accidents. There are also problems for the children of depressed parents; they are more vulnerable to emotional and cognitive impairment, which in turn can predispose to adult mental illness on maturity, as well as having an adverse effect on the children's ultimate intellectual attainment. Chronic non-psychotic illness such as chronic depression, persistent unresolved grief states, chronic phobias, and tranquilliser dependency leads not only to considerable stress, and a low quality of life, but also may act as a trigger for alcohol and drug abuse, excessive burden on health services, as well as a loss of productive economic activity.

As long ago as 1973, the World Health Organisation listed some of the other major reasons why it considered that the GP is best placed to deal with the primary care of mental illness[2]. First, very many of the mentally ill present with a physical complaint and do not consider themselves to be in need of psychiatric care. Secondly, physical and mental illness frequently co-exist. Doctors used to be trained to diagnose only one illness in a patient rather than several, and there is evidence that psychiatrists frequently miss physical disorder, while GPs and other physicians often miss psychiatric disorder. Thus exclusive preoccupation with one specialty may be disastrous for the individual patient. Thirdly, many psychiatric disorders are connected with family problems and social difficulties, and are only understandable when viewed against this background. The good GP may carry much of this in his or her head while the psychiatrist has to spend valuable time obtaining the relevant information. And lastly, GPs are well placed to provide long term follow up and support.

Prevention

The particular focus of this conference on depression and anxiety is prevention. A good prevention strategy should not be a small addition to our daily work, done only when time allows. Rather it should be an integral part of a comprehensive health care service.

Responsibility for the prevention of illness and promotion of health care should be shared; between individuals, families, informal support networks, voluntary organisations, primary and secondary health care professionals and the Government. All of us must work together to create a health care system which promotes the health of the nation and the health of individuals – as well as treating existing disorders. The prevention of mental illness is of particular importance because of the very heavy burdens it imposes – not only on the people who suffer from mental illness, but also, on their families, and on the primary and secondary care services.

Mental illness has very significant economic implications nationally. In 1989, Caroline Croft-Jeffreys and Greg Wilkinson estimated the cost of depression and anxiety (including lost production) at up to £5.6 billion/year[3]. As these are the commonest forms of mental illness found in the United Kingdom, it seemed appropriate to hold this conference on their prevention. The *Primary Care of Schizophrenia* followed[4].

I would like in closing, therefore, to thank everyone who contributed to the meeting and to the book. My thanks would not be complete without giving mention to the four chairmen who so skilfully managed their sessions and stimulated valuable discussion, much of which is reflected in these pages.

Thank you: Michael Shepherd CBE, Emeritus Professor of Epidemiological Psychiatry, Institute of Psychiatry, London; Stuart Carne CBE, President, The Royal College of General Practitioners; Mollie McBride, Honorary Secretary, The Royal College of General Practitioners; and Colin Waine, Vice Chairman of the Council of The Royal College of Practitioners. (Positions as at March 1990).

Address for contact

Dr J L Reed, Senior Principal Medical Officer, Department of Health, Health Care (Medical) Division, Wellington House, 133–155 Waterloo Road, London SE1 8UG

References

1. Department of Health. *Caring for people: community care in the next decade and beyond*. London: HMSO, 1989 Cm 849
2. World Health Organisation 1973, Psychiatry and Primary Medical Care, WHO, Copenhagen
3. Croft-Jeffries C, Wilkinson G. Estimated costs of neurotic disorders in UK general practice in 1985. *Psychol Med* 1989 **19** 549–558
4. Jenkins R, Field V and Young R. The primary care of schizophrenia. London, HMSO 1992

Foreword B

DR COLIN WAINE, OBE, FRCGP Chairman of Council, Royal College of General Practitioners

The general practitioner is in a unique position to play a key role in the prevention of depression and anxiety. He or she frequently has contact with their patients and their patients families, over a long period of time, and gains an intimate knowledge of their physical, psychological and social problems.

Psychological problems are prominent in about a quarter of consultations with adults in general practice and psychosocial factors are present to a significant degree in about half of consultations concerning children.

In February 1981, the Royal College of General Practitioners published *prevention of Psychiatric Disorder in General Practice*. In that document, it was acknowledged that a preventive strategy had not yet been developed to tackle what was recognised as an enormous part of the workload of a general practitioner. It recognised the dearth of relevant research but attempted to use that which was available to develop a preventive approach. Furthermore it succeeded in challenging general practice, primary care and psychiatry to begin to think in preventive terms.

The 15–16 March 1990 saw a notable coming together of the Department of Health, the Prevention Project of MIND and the Royal College of General Practitioners at a conference 'Prevention of Depression and Anxiety – The Role of the Practice Team'.

This important conference was held at the Royal College of Physicians, London. The fact that on each of the two days the large lecture theatre was virtually filled to capacity was, I believe, an expression of the importance that delegates attach to trying to prevent these two most distressing conditions which figure so prominently in general practice.

This publication is based on the presentations given at that conference, which have kindly been brought together under the editorship of Dr Robyn Young. It will be of great value not only to general practitioners and primary care teams, but very importantly, to those members of the primary care team at present in training.

It is a privilege for me to write this foreword and thereby to be allowed to link my name to those of the distinguished contributors in the search for better ways of preventing the distress and suffering caused by anxiety and depression.

Reference

Prevention of Psychiatric Disorders in General Practice. Report from General Practice No 20, London, Royal College of General Practitioners, 1981.

1 Depression and Anxiety in Primary Care: The Epidemiological Evidence

ANTHONY MANN, Professor of Epidemiological Psychiatry, Institute of Psychiatry, London

SUMMARY

The non-psychotic psychiatric disorders of primary care, largely symptoms of anxiety and depression, are a major health problem: a source of much personal distress, chronic morbidity and economic cost. The occurrence and outcome of these illnesses are influenced by the quality of family and marital relationships and other social support networks. Non-medical interventions which enable people to develop more satisfying personal and social contacts would help decrease the prevalence of these illnesses and relieve the growing burden on general practice.

Introduction

Family doctors: the first port of call

Approximately 60–70 per cent of the adult population will at some time experience depression or worry of sufficient severity to influence their daily activities. There is a great variation in individual tolerance, but the episodes are mostly short-lived, related to life events, and they pass. However, for some, the experience is much more severe and alarming. The symptoms persist. Sufferers feel low-spirited, with a loss of energy and enjoyment. They worry, cannot sleep or concentrate, and often experience physical symptoms which become a source of considerable concern. Quality of life and competence to manage are impaired.

Some people tolerate this distress; others seek help. In Britain, the first port of call is usually the family doctor, not a specialist psychologist or psychiatrist, as might be the case in other countries. In fact, many people who feel anxious or depressed in this way would be upset if asked to see a psychiatrist. Whether they choose to consult a doctor will depend on several personal concepts: their views about what illness is; when it is appropriate to see a doctor; how ill they believe themselves to be compared with their normal selves. At consultation, the general practitioner (GP) tries to formulate what is wrong – according to his or her diagnostic framework; applies a diagnostic label; and then tries to help. The psychiatrist is in the background, seeing such patients only at the GP's request.

Research carried out over the last 25 years by colleagues at the Institute of Psychiatry's General Practice Research Unit, directed by Professor Michael Shepherd, has shown that consultations for anxiety and depression form a significant part of the GP's day-to-day case load. These conditions can be as chronic and as severe as many of those seen by psychiatrists (see also Chapter 3) and prove expensive for the Health Service.

Two major barriers bedevil the understanding of these disorders and interfere with the relationships between patient and family doctor, and family doctor and psychiatrist:

(i) *'Neurosis':* Until the recent promotion of changes in terminology (originating from the United States), persistent depressed or anxious states received a diagnostic label from the GP or psychiatrist of anxiety or depressive 'neurosis'. The adjective 'neurotic', in lay terms, has come to imply complaining, or attention-seeking people. In clinical use, anxiety and depressive 'neurosis' are technical terms which describe a group of psychiatric syndromes – no value judgement is or should be implied.

(ii) **Attribution:** People feeling depressed or anxious often seek explanations for this state in their personal circumstances: for to be anxious or depressed for no reason is hard to accept. They then present their reasons (attribution) to their GP who may come to share their perspective. The doctor understands the problems and pressures bearing upon the patient, whether these be adverse social circumstances or painful, physical illness. Depression may be seen as part and parcel of the circumstances and therefore not to be treated as a condition in its own right. In contrast, a psychiatrist is more likely to pay attention to the severity and extent of symptoms and functional disability and treats these independent of the cause. A difference in perspective thus often exists between psychiatrists consulting or carrying out research within general practice and GPs themselves.

The scale of the problem

Table 1.1 shows the comparative rates of attendance for different levels of psychiatric care in England and Wales in 1981.

Table 1.1: *Comparative rates of attendance for different levels of psychiatric care (rates per 100,000 general population England and Wales, all ages and sexes combined) in 1981*

	General practitioner consultations[1]	Outpatient attendances[2]	Day hospital attendances[2]	Psychiatric admissions[2]
ICD-9 290–315 Mental disorders	22,980	2,532	4,943	397

Source:
1: Morbidity Statistics from General practice **1981–1982**, Third National Study, RCGP, OPCS, DHSS
2: Mental Health Enquiry for England, 1981

Table based on: Sharp D and Morrell D (1989). See reference 1.

The number of contacts reported for psychiatric disorder in primary care is more than twice the total recorded for all forms of specialist psychiatric contact[1]. National Morbidity Statistics for 1981 (ie, for England and Wales) show that, at 9 per cent, psychiatric disorders are the third most common cause of consultation in primary care, following those concerning (i) the respiratory system (15 per cent); and (ii) the cardiovascular system (11 per cent). It has long been established – for example, by Shepherd's cardinal study in 1966[2] (Table 1.2) and by reports such as that of the Royal College of General Practitioners in 1973 (Table 1.3)[3] – that the non-psychotic psychiatric disorders (largely anxiety and depression) form the bulk of the GP's psychiatric workload.

Table 1.2: *Patient consulting rates per 1,000 persons registered with a GP, at risk for psychiatric morbidity by sex and diagnostic group*

Diagnostic group	Male	Female	Both sexes
Psychoses	2.7	8.6	5.0
Mental subnormality	1.6	2.9	2.3
Dementia	1.2	1.6	1.4
Neuroses	55.7	116.6	88.5
Personality disorder	7.2	4.0	5.5
Formal psychiatric illness*	67.2	131.9	102.1
Psychosomatic conditions	24.5	34.5	29.9
Organic illness with psychiatric overlay	13.1	16.6	15.0
Psychosocial problems	4.6	10.0	7.5
Psychiatric-associated conditions*	38.6	57.2	48.6
Total psychiatric morbidity*	97.9	175.0	139.4
Number of patients at risk	6,783	7,914	14,697

* These totals cannot be obtained by adding the rates for the relevant diagnostic groups because while a pateint may be included in more than one diagnostic group, he will be included only once in the total. Shepherd et al 1966[2]

Table 1.3: *Psychiatric disorder and social pathology in an average general practice population of 2,500*

Acute major disorders	Cases per annum
Severe depression	12
Suicide attempts	3
Completed suicide	One very three years
Chronic mental illness	55
Severe mental handicap	10
Neurotic disorders	300

Social pathology

Chronic alcoholism (known cases)	
Chronic alcoholism (unkown cases)	25
Juvenile delinquency	5–7
Problem families	5–10
Broken homes (one-parent families with children under 15)	60

Source: Royal College of General Practitioners (1973). See reference 3.

The 'Walking Worried'?

Research among GP consulters, regardless of whether they are also physically ill, indicates that over a third are in total or in part suffering from psychiatric disorder. It is pertinent to ask whether these patients are really *ill?* or warrant the costly attention given by health-care professionals or indeed, extensive research. Critics dismiss these complaints as minor psychiatric syndromes, and have described the patients themselves as the *'walking worried'*.

Three types of evidence counter such dismissive views and indicate that these disorders can pose major problems for both the providers of health care and the patients themselves:

(i) *Clinical studies* have compared the symptomatology of states of depression and anxiety found in hospital with those seen in general practice: few differences have emerged[4]. Very severely depressed patients are usually referred to specialist clinics, a fact which could persuade hospital psychiatrists that the conditions they are seeing are different to those presenting in general practice. However, many severe depressions are found in general practice, where they make up at least five per cent of all consultations for psychiatric disorders[5]. The association between successful suicide and recent consultation with a family doctor also indicates that very severely depressed people do seek help from that source[6].

(ii) *Treatment* of these conditions shows that GPs seem to regard some form of medication as necessary. Figure 1.1 shows the volume of prescriptions for psychotropic drugs dispensed by retail pharmacies throughout England between the late 1960s and 1970s. Table 1.4 gives an interesting snapshot of more recent prescribing habits on a smaller scale: of the prescriptions for the same category of drugs issued by four GPs in a city suburban practice over a one-week period in January 1983. Psychotropic drugs were the commonest form of medication prescribed and accounted for roughly 30 per cent of the total first and repeat prescriptions issued during that week.

Table 1.4: *A profile of psychotropic drugs[1] prescribed during one week by a 4-man general practice, London 1983*

Psychotropic drug	Prescriptions (Percentage of total)	
	Initial	Repeat
Tranquillisers	32	26
% Minor	60	70
% Major	30	22
% Methadone	10	8
Hypnotics	19	33
Antidepressants	10	8
Analgesics	16	8
Other	13	25
Stimulants	3	0

[1] The commonest category of drugs prescribed during the one-week period.
Source: Mann A H. Study of psychiatric attachment in general practice (in preparation).

Figure 1.1 *Prescriptions dispensed at retail pharmacies in England 1966–1977 and 1987*

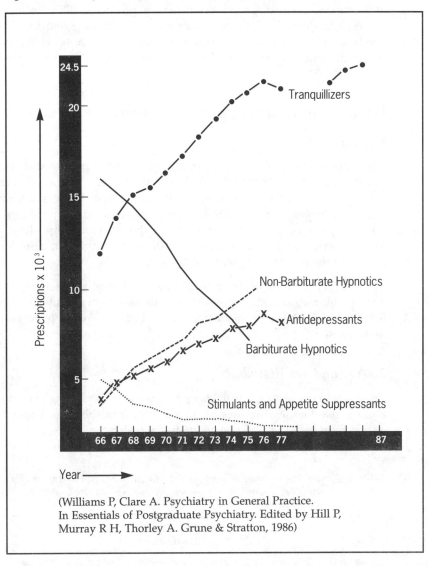

(Williams P, Clare A. Psychiatry in General Practice. In Essentials of Postgraduate Psychiatry. Edited by Hill P, Murray R H, Thorley A. Grune & Stratton, 1986)

Table 1.5: *Cost of neurotic disorder in general practice in the United Kingdom, 1985*

Item	Costs (£ million)
Consultations } General practice	119.5
Drugs	
Sickness absence	253
TOTAL (minimal estimate)	372.5
Plus	
Early retirement	2,700
Uncertified sickness absence	2,900
TOTAL	5,600

Source: Based on Croft-Jeffreys C, and & Wilkinson G (1989). See reference 7.

(iii) *Costs*: In 1989, Croft-Jeffreys and Wilkinson calculated the economic costs of the non-psychotic disorders seen in general practice in 1985, throughout the United Kingdom. They costed the expenses of the time and the treatment involved, and estimated the impact of these disorders upon the patients' economic functioning[7]. The total, as seen in Table 1.5, approached £6,000,000,000.

What is known about these psychiatric disorders?

1. Prevalence

It is important to emphasise that the centrally collected published statistics, for example the National Morbidity Statistics from General Practice, concern only those people recognised by the GP at consultation to be suffering from significant psychiatric disorder. Goldberg and other colleagues[8] introduced the concepts of (i) *conspicuous morbidity* – ie, the psychiatric disorder is known to the practitioner; and (ii) *hidden morbidity* ie, the psychiatric disorder is not known to the practitioner (see Chapter 4).

The proportion is approximately 2:1, but obviously varies from doctor to doctor. This means that the prevalence of these disorders is much larger than the National Morbidity Statistics show, because many patients remain undiagnosed.

2. Age and sex distribution

The age and sex of a typical 100 people consulting GPs in England and Wales and the psychiatric diagnoses by the GP appear in Table 1.6. These data are drawn from the 1974 National Morbidity Statistics.[9]

Table 1.6: *The composition of a cohort calculated to be representative of patients attending general practitioners with non-psychotic psychiatric disorders in England and Wales*

	GP's diagnosis									Psychiatrist's diagnosis
	Age in years									
	Women (N=72)				Men (N=28)					
	15–24	25–44	45–64	65+	15–24	25–44	45–64	65+	**TOTAL**	**TOTAL**
Anxiety neurosis/ phobic neurosis	3	9	8	3	1	4	4	1	33	33
Depressive neurosis	3	11	10	5	1	3	4	1	38	56
Physical disorders of psychogenic origin/tension headache	2	5	4	1	1	2	2	0	17	3
Insomnia	0	1	1	1	0	0	1	1	5	2
Other conditions	1	2	1	1	0	1	1	0	7	6
TOTAL	9	28	24	11	3	10	12	3	100	100

Source: OPCS National Morbidity Statistics (1974) HMSO[9]. See reference 13

The commonest diagnoses were anxiety and depression and, in women, the commonest age-group was the 25 to 44-year-olds. The results probably underestimate the number of patients in the older age-groups (>65 years) as these figures are based upon conspicuous morbidity, and psychiatric syndromes are often not diagnosed in older people. For instance, a survey carried out in 1988[10], amongst 813 elderly men and women of pensionable age resident in North London, found that some 16 per cent were clinically depressed, 36 per cent of them having depressive symptoms. Half of the former had consulted their GP in the preceeding month, but only one in eight of them had received anti-depressant medication. Prescription of anti-depressants could have been reduced by factors such as the presence of ischaemic heart disease, but there was no evidence that any other action had been taken to relieve the depression.

The sex difference is noticeable. Approximately two and a half times as many women consult GPs as do men. This difference has remained remarkably stable throughout all general practice research studies[11].

3. *Comparison of GP and psychiatrist diagnoses*

Table 1.6 also shows a comparison of the GPs' diagnoses of psychiatric disorders seen in primary care with those of the psychiatrist who independently interviewed the same patients. Psychiatrists tend to diagnose more depression than GPs: physical disorders of psychogenic origin and insomnia being categories that contribute to this discrepancy.

4. *Association with*

(a) Physical illness

Anxiety and depression are associated both at the time of presentation and during the lifetime of an individual, with the presence of physical illness. Eastwood and Trevelyan 1972[12], first showed that clustering of both psychiatric and physical illnesses tends to occur in the same individuals. This has been confirmed in other cross-section and longitudinal studies (see also Chapter 2). The implications of this association are that:

(i) Psychiatric disorders are often missed in primary care practice because the co-existing physical disease dominates the diagnosis;
(ii) Management of the psychiatric state must take physical status into account; and
(iii) There is an important implication for the understanding of the genesis of these disorders. There seems to be a psycho-physiological process at work, rather than a purely psychological one.

(b) Social adversity

A strong relationship exists with social adversity (see also Chapter 3). Patients seen in primary care with depression and anxiety show much more evidence of social stress – eg, limited and difficult personal relationships; less satisfaction with their occupation and other practical aspects of daily life. This has implications for the prediction, prevention and management of anxiety and depression.

Outcome

Those who wish to minimise the need for resources for anxiety/depressive disorders claim that patients recover any way. Indeed, little research has been done on their natural history in primary care, but it is known that only five per cent of these patients are referred for specialist help[8]. Of the remainder, the general clinical impression is that while most episodes clear up, a significant proportion of patients suffer a protracted illness (see also Chapter 3). To this end, a one-year follow-up study was carried out in Warwickshire, of 100 patients found by their GP to be suffering from neurotic illness and, by dint of their age, sex and diagnosis, considered to be representative of patients with neurotic illness consulting GPs throughout England[13]. A typical cohort was drawn and received detailed initial assessment, monitoring of contact with the general practice over the following year, and reassessment at the end of that year. The psychiatrists assessed the patients' psychiatric symptoms, their perceived stresses and supports in the social environment, and their personality (as reported at interview by an informant).

One year later, 50 per cent of the patients had recovered. Factors present at the initial assessment which predicted a poor outcome:

(i) A severe initial symptom state.
(ii) The patient's perception of a poor quality of social life or of marital support.
(iii) Prescription of a psychotropic drug by the GP during the year of follow-up.

Analysis of the course of these disorders over the intervening year showed that approximately 25 per cent of the patients recovered in the first months of the follow-up year and did not relapse; about 50 per cent had intermittent relapses; and 25 per cent ran a chronic course with apparently regular consultations and perpetual complaints of psychiatric symptoms. Factors assessed at the beginning of the follow-up year which were associated with membership of these outcome groups are shown in Table 1.7.

Table 1.7: *Course of neurotic illness over 12 months in general practice[1]*

Patients		
Group A	Rapid improvement	24%
Group B	Intermittent relapses	52%
Group C	Chronic course	25%

Predictors of rapid improvement: A vs B and C (p<.01)
Perceived good family support year 1
Perceived good social support year 2
No psychotropic medication

Predictors of chronic course: C vs A and B (p<.01)
High overall severity score (psychiatric) year 1
Presence of physical illness year 2
Receipt of psychotropic drugs

[1]Source: Mann A H, Jenkins R and Belsey E (1981) See reference 13

Conclusion

The non-psychotic disorders of primary care, largely anxiety and depression, are the source of much personal distress, chronic morbidity and economic cost in the UK. Even in a prosperous area of the country, a quarter of the people consulting their GP for depression developed a chronic illness with continuous complaints, regular consultation and poor outcome one year later. This chronic sub-group, increasingly well-recognised both here and in the United States, is placing a constant load on GPs. The best indicators for a rapid recovery includes the patient's perception of having good support from their marriage, the family and local social networks.

References

1. Sharp D, Morrell D. *The psychiatry of general practice*. In: Williams P, Wilkinson G, Rawnsley K, editors. The scope of epidemiological psychiatry. London: Routledge, 1989: 404–419.

2. Shepherd M, Cooper B, Brown A C, Kalton G W. *Psychiatric illness in general practice*. London: Oxford University Press, 1966.

3. Royal College of General Practitioners. *Present status and future needs of general practice*. London: Royal College of General Practitioners, 1973. (Reports on general practice no 16).

4. Brown G W, Craig T K J, Harris T O. Depression: disease or distress? Some epidemiological considerations. *Br J Psychiatry* 1985;**147**:612–622.

5. Blacker C V R, Clare A W. Depressive disorder in primary care. *Br J Psychiatry* 1987;**150**:737–751.

6. Barraclough B, Bunch J, Nelson B, Sainsbury P. A hundred cases of suicide: clinical aspects. *Br J Psychiatry* 1974;**125**:355–373.

7. Croft-Jeffreys C, Wilkinson G. Estimated costs of neurotic disorder in the UK general practice 1985. *Psychol Med* 1989;**19**:549–558.

8. Goldberg D P, Huxley P. *Mental illness in the community: the pathway to psychiatric care*. London: Tavistock, 1980.

9. Office of Population Censuses and Surveys. *Morbidity statistics from general practice: second national study 1970–71*. London: Office of Population Censuses and Surveys, 1974. (Studies on medical and population subject: 26).

10. Livingston G, Hawkins A, Graham N, Blizard R, Mann A H. The Gospel Oak Study: prevalence rates of dementia, depression and activity limitation among elderly residents in Inner London. *Psychol Med* 1990;**20**:137–146.

11. Briscoe M. Sex difference in psychological well-being. *Psychol Med Monogr Suppl* 1982;**1**.

12. Eastwood M R, Tevelyan M H. Relationship between physical and psychiatric disorder. *Psychol Med* 1972;**2**:363–372.

13. Mann A, Jenkins R, Belsey E. The twelve-month outcome of patients with neurotic illness in general practice. *Psychol Med* 1981;**11**:535–550.

Further Reading

Goldberg D P, Huxley P. *Mental illness in the community: the pathway to psychiatric care*. London: Tavistock, 1980.

Shepherd M, Clare A. *Psychiatric illness in general practice*. Oxford: Oxford University Press, second edition 1981.

Address for contact

Professor Anthony Mann, Section of Epidemiology and General Practice, Institute of Psychiatry, De Crespigny Park, London SE5 8AF.

2 Depression and Anxiety: An overview of Preventive Strategies

RACHEL JENKINS, Principal Medical Officer,
Department of Health, London

SUMMARY

Depression and anxiety place enormous burdens on people and resources throughout the United Kingdom. Early detection and treatment offer a good prognosis, and prevention is increasingly possible. Primary care has a crucial role to play in implementing prevention strategies. This paper briefly reviews the prevalence of depression and anxiety and, using the scheme of primary, secondary and tertiary prevention, describes strategies for prevention based upon a clear understanding of the risk factors which cause and prolong the illness. The importance of education about prevention is highlighted, both for the general population, and also for undergraduate and postgraduate doctors, who need to learn about the relationships between physical and psychological illness, the principles of multiaxial assessment, and the role of multidisciplinary liaison in detection and management of these disorders.

Background: Why prevention deserves priority

Unrecognised or inadequately-treated psychological illnesses take a severe toll of the quality and the length of life of millions of people. Population surveys, as indicated by Professor Mann, estimate prevalence rates of 2–3 per cent for the functional psychoses, and 15–25 per cent for the non-psychotic disorders of depression and anxiety and other neuroses. Depression and anxiety are, in fact, the commonest psychological disorders diagnosed in the United Kingdom and are among the top few of all the illnesses seen in general practice[1]. The cumulative economic burden caused by these disorders, in terms of lost productivity, absence due to sickness, labour turnover, accidents, and medical care is enormous; the cost in human suffering, incalculable. Data which give some indication of marital breakdown and violence, cognitive damage to children, and the number of children placed in care, only hint at the extent of the problem.

In 1986, the 39th World Health Assembly called on Member States (which includes us!) to include preventive measures, identified by the World Health Organisation (WHO)[2], in their national health strategies and, by then applying these measures, to achieve *'Health for All by the Year 2000'*. Each country was also asked to organise appropriate training programmes for health workers and to stimulate, co-ordinate and conduct research on prevention.

A working definition for prevention

In 1964, Caplan[3] divided prevention into *primary, secondary* and *tertiary* activities:

Primary prevention refers to methods designed to avoid the occurrence of disease; ie, it prevents the *incidence* of mental disorder by counteracting adverse factors before they can cause a disorder. For example, a balanced diet will prevent dementia caused by pellagra (nicotinic acid deficiency); measles immunisation prevents mental retardation caused by measles encephalitis.

Secondary prevention refers to early diagnosis and treatment which shorten the length of episodes of illness, minimise the chances of transmission, and limit the adverse consequences of the illness. Secondary prevention aims to *reduce the prevalence* of mental disorder. The timely treatment of one condition can also have primary preventive effects on others. For example, the detection and management of hypertension helps prevent cerebrovascular disease, strokes and arteriosclerotic dementia; the control of epilepsy reduces the number of accidents and work injuries.

Tertiary prevention refers to measures which *limit disability* and handicap caused by an illness which might not itself be fully treatable. For example, adequate rehabilitation facilities in the community help prevent deterioration in schizophrenia[4] or mental handicap[5]. It is often not so much the disease per se, but how the health care system responds, which determines the extent of a patient's disability.

Primary prevention is claimed, by some, to be the only *real* prevention. Secondary and tertiary prevention are said to be 'just good practice' – examples of efficient diagnosis and management. Such views ignore many possibilities for action and improvement. Secondary and tertiary prevention can dramatically improve detection and recovery rates, reduce disability, and have a primary preventive effect on other knock-on consequences of mental illness. Developing strategies for secondary and tertiary prevention also encourages clinicians to look for *hidden morbidity*, as well as apply good practice to *conspicuous cases* (see Chapter 4).

Prevention requires a clear understanding of the aetiology, pathogenesis, and natural progression of an illness. Knowledge of risk factors points the way to effective prevention strategies (see Chapter 8). Populations with a greater-than-average risk of certain illnesses can and must be identified.

Causes of depression

It is helpful to think of aetiological factors in mental illness (including depression) as:

1. Predisposing,
2. Precipitating, and
3. Maintaining[6].

Each factor can also have:
   a. Biological
   b. Social and
   c. Psychological components.

1. *Predisposing factors* increase *vulnerability* to a particular illness in the future.

a. ***Biological*** *predisposing factors* include: genetic constitution (ie, what we inherit); intrauterine damage (eg, alcohol, cigarette smoke and other toxins); birth trauma (eg, brain injury); and physical deprivation in childhood.

b. ***Social*** *predisposing factors* include: emotional deprivation in childhood (including being 'in care'); bereavement or separation – particularly from parents or spouse; chronic work or marital difficulties; and lack of supportive personal and social relationships.

c. ***Psychological*** *predisposing factors* include: poor parental role models (eg, of violence or mental illness); excessive illness behaviour (eg, withdrawal from normal role activities); low self-esteem – particularly in women; and learned helplessness. A helpless approach to life can be learnt by people whose past experience has led them to believe that their own actions *cannot* influence their circumstances (see also Chapter 3).

2. *Precipitating factors* determine when the illness starts.

a. ***Biological*** *precipitating factors* include: recent infections, disabling injury, and malignant disease.

b. ***Social*** *precipitating factors* include: recent life events – particularly those which involve the threat of, or actual loss. Redundancy, unemployment, major illness in the family, a child leaving home, separation or divorce, and the loss of a supportive relationship are common examples of life events preceding illness.

c. ***Psychological*** *precipitating factors* refer to inappropriate responses, to the biological and social factors above. These 'maladjustments' evoke feelings of helplessness and hopelessness in the person concerned.

3. *Maintaining factors* *prolong* an illness and *delay* recovery.

a. ***Biological*** *maintaining factors* include: chronic pain or disability. Special note should be made of sensory disability – eg, the loss of sight or hearing – which puts individuals at a particular disadvantage.

b. ***Social*** *maintaining factors* include: chronic social stresses and pressures related to problems with housing, finance, work, marriage, family and friends; and, more specifically – lack of an intimate, confiding relationship at home, or support from colleagues and friends; and lack of practical information about how to deal with social problems, overcome and manage psychological difficulties, and find sources of practical help.

c. ***Psychological*** *maintaining factors* include: low self-esteem, doubts about personal recovery from illness, and the effects of *welfare dependency*. This latter type of behaviour seems to run in certain families which, from one generation to another, are well know to all the caring agencies – especially social workers –

accruing enormous files in Social Services departments and general practice records.

Primary prevention of depression and anxiety

Depression and anxiety can afflict anyone. Some measures of primary prevention are therefore relevant for the *whole population*, while others are more usefully targeted at groups who are at particularly *high risk*. Thus, primary prevention may be categorised into universal measures, selective measures and indicated measures.

(i) *Universal* measures: directed at the *whole population* – eg, health education, immunisation, good nutrition, stopping smoking, dental hygiene, and the use of seat belts.

(ii) *Selective* measures: recommended for relatively *large sub-groups* whose risk of becoming ill is 'above normal': eg, the avoidance of alcohol and non-essential medications by pregnant women.

(iii) *Indicated* measures: for relatively *small sub-groups* considered to be at sufficiently-high risk to require the preventive intervention – eg, support for an isolated, blind, disabled, elderly man who has lost his spouse.

It is also helpful to relate prevention strategies to recognised developmental stages in the life cycle. These stages may then be chosen for special intervention. A brief look at early stages in a life-cycle approach follows, and Caryle Steen describes how it may be implemented in general practice, in Chapter 14.

Universal measures eg educating children and adolescents

This issue, although not strictly belonging to the start of the life-cycle prevention model, is fundamental to success. Children and adolescents need to develop a core of stored knowledge and basic understanding about physical and psychological development and personal needs: about the relevance of good nutrition, the risks of teenage pregnancies, the importance of good parenting skills, and the nature and value of social networks. It is also important to help them develop constructive attitudes towards mental illness – including its treatability and to understand the need to combat stigma. Such knowledge can help young people pass from childhood dependence to adult life more successfully; encourage them to take part in health-promoting activities such as those outlined below; and so provide a sound basis for their own, and future dependants', physical and mental health. These issues have now been developed and incorporated into National Curriculum Guidance V[7].

Selective measures of preconception, prenatal and perinatal care

People planning to start a family need information about nutrition; about the avoidance of smoking, alcohol and drugs in the period leading up to conception; and about environmental hazards which affect foetal development.

Prenatal care should involve both parents wherever possible, and aim to provide optimum conditions for foetal development. High-risk pregnancies should be recognised, and efforts taken to prevent prematurity and low-birthweight babies. Work by Cutting[8] shows that reducing the risk of intra-uterine damage and birth trauma reduces vulnerability to mental illness in later life: Murray and colleagues have linked the falling incidence of schizophrenia in postwar years to improved perinatal care[9].

Pregnant women and their partners or, as may be the case with single mothers-to-be, their families, need ready access to expert obstetric care and advice on issues fundamental to their own and the unborn infant's immediate and long-term health[10]. Topics of prime importance include:

(i) *Nutrition:* The relationship between good nutrition and healthy foetal growth – including cognitive development – should be explained, special attention being given to high-risk groups – eg, low-income families, the unemployed, the homeless, and certain ethnic minority groups. Advice must take into account factors such as limited financial resources and different cultural beliefs and practices.

(ii) *Breast feeding* should be encouraged: eg, by explaining its major advantages, and by providing help to establish the practice – in hospital after the birth, and on returning home.

(iii) *Tobacco smoking and the use of alcohol and illegal drugs*, should be discussed routinely, together with *prescribed and self-administered* (over-the-counter) *medications*. The harm they can cause to the unborn child, as well as the mother, is often poorly understood. Common problems, such as the harmful effects of passive smoking on the newborn baby, other young children and members of the family, should be highlighted; support for giving up smoking should be offered. The use of shared syringes by injecting drug users, and the associated dangers of HIV virus transmission is an essential topic for high-risk groups. The importance of discussing any proposed medication with the GP in the light of the pregnancy should be emphasised.

(iv) *'Immunisation'* is a topic suitable for antenatal courses. Parents thus prepared should more readily comply with schedules recommended for their infants by their family practice. The decrease in mental handicap, as well as physical birth defects, associated with the popular acceptance of rubella immunisation, and similarly, the decrease in measles encephalitis as a result of measles immunisation are two excellent examples of successful primary prevention strategies.

(v) *Relaxation and stress-reduction techniques* can provide welcome benefit to parents and child carers – particularly single parents and those without close relatives or other family support.

(vi) *Child health and development* can also be introduced into prenatal courses and its study continued, with help from the primary care team, throughout the infant and pre-school period. Parents should be made aware of their child's psychological needs as well as of stages in his or her physical development.

(vii) *Playing:* Children who play with their parents, as well as with their toys and friends, are much more likely to grow up socially well-adjusted and less vulnerable to adult depression[10]. The child who plays frequently also develops better language skills more rapidly – a very important asset and developmental milestone.

15

(viii) *Safety:* Children need a safe environment to play in – one free from traffic and molestation. Accidents are the commonest cause of death in children aged one year: pedestrian deaths form a significant component of the total[11].

Indicated Measures eg (a) Social support for at-risk groups

Although some life events and chronic social stresses can be avoided by careful planning, many occur as unpredicted crises or 'Acts of God'. Social support networks buffer the effects of acute and chronic stress and help prevent or shorten the duration of depression and anxiety[12,13,14]. Social support need not require complicated or expensive action. Just someone to talk to, or someone who will listen to your problems can be sufficient. George Brown highlights the importance of supportive relationships in Chapter 3; and indeed, it receives frequent mention throughout this book.

In an ideal world, everyone would have adequate personal networks from which to obtain support in times of need. In real life, these networks are often lacking, and although GPs should not be expected to fill the gap, they should be able to mobilise members of their practice team, choosing whoever seems appropriate for a particular task. Self help groups, voluntary agencies, trained counsellors, practice and district nurses, health visitors, attached psychologists and social workers, the local authority social workers should be called upon to help as necessary.

Support should be offered to *at-risk* groups after major life events such as bereavement[15], redundancy[16] and retirement. The intervention should come as soon as possible after the event(s), or even before, if the event can be anticipated (eg, retirement, redundancy, parenthood). Individual counselling is often appropriate for bereavement, but group counselling may be more appropriate for people approaching redundancy and retirement.

Childbirth is a major life event which can impose stress upon the marital relationship, and foster anxiety, through chronic sleeplessness and fatigue. Many mothers who have left work to look after their child become socially isolated, intellectually unstimulated, and so, depressed. On the other hand, mothers who return promptly to work can find themselves overstretched and exhausted – with no time to 'recharge their batteries'. For many women, befriending support groups such as Newpin and Home-Start can provide essential help (see Chapter 13).

(b) Treatment of physical disease

Depression and anxiety often occur as a secondary consequence of blindness, deafness, immobility, or physical disease – particularly progressive, painful, or life-threatening conditions: eg, multiple sclerosis, rheumatoid arthritis and cancer. They can also be symptoms of physical illnesses such as endocrine disorders, viral or bacterial infections. The early detection and treatment of sensory deficits, physical disease and immobility, will greatly reduce the risk of depression.

*(c) **The Elderly*** with their increased chances of physical disease, sensory deficits, immobility and social isolation, are particularly at risk for depression and suicide.

(d) Treatment of mental illness in parents

Mental illness in parents can cause physical and emotional deprivation in children, and so predispose them to mental illness in adult life. Rutter and Madge called this sequence of events the *Cycle of Disadvantage*[17], a description which highlights the relevance of preventive action – ie, the ability of the early detection and treatment of depression and anxiety to avert immediate and long-term harmful effects.

Children whose parents are suffering from mental illness need special attention and support. Well-meaning, but poorly-informed adult friends will often offer children strange and guarded advice; the children might find themselves quite incapable of understanding their parent's changed or erratic behaviour; and there may be difficulties in the school setting. Children tend to blame themselves for their parents' behaviour, and therefore skilled support, understanding, and explanation are needed to protect the child against long-term psychological damage.

These parents also need social support – someone to share their experiences; someone who can, for example, offer occasional, practical relief such as baby-sitting. This support is crucial for single parents and couples who have no extended family.

Secondary prevention of depression and anxiety

Early detection and treatment

Depression frequently goes unrecognised and remains untreated[18] (see Chapter 4). Untreated depression is associated with an increased risk of physical illness (and hence, increased morbidity and mortality), suicide and para-suicide, marital breakdown, poor parenting, and occupational problems – such as sickness absence, high labour turnover, problems with colleagues, poor performance, and accidents[19]. As we have seen, it also causes emotional and cognitive impairment in children. However, if treated, depression has a good prognosis and responds well to supportive measures – including counselling and antidepressant medication[20,21]. Anxiety responds to relaxation techniques and behaviour management. Early diagnosis and appropriate management are therefore extremely important.

Who should do the detecting?

Depression and anxiety occur in about one in three of the patients attending general practice. Studies show that GPs detect only about half (***conspicuous morbidity***) and miss about half (***hidden morbidity***) of these patients[18]. Detection of patients in the hidden morbidity group improves their prognosis significantly[22].

GPs and members of the primary care team have key roles in the detection, assessment and management of both depression and anxiety. They need to be trained for this task, and the composition of the primary care team needs to be developed to cope with depression at all stages of the life cycle. Linda Gask (see Chapter 5) and Paul Freeling (see Chapter 7) emphasise the importance of interview skills and self-knowledge in the detection of depression. The team also needs skills in supportive counselling, the use of antidepressants for depression, and behaviour therapy for anxiety.

GP time is limited, so it would seem appropriate that much essential psychosocial intervention should be delegated to appropriate members of the team – eg, to counsellors, attached social workers and psychologists, primary care nurses (including practice and district nurses), and health visitors. All these professional groups can play a key role in detecting depression. For example, health visitors are best placed to detect depression in young, isolated mothers of pre-school children; district nurses are best placed to diagnose depression in the elderly. Social Services personnel, such as domiciliary care workers are also in close contact with elderly people, and with clients who have long-term physical and sensory disabilities.

Undergraduate and continuing medical education

Professor Freeling discusses the importance of undergraduate and continuing medical education – particularly as it affects GPs – in Chapter 7. I wish to emphasise the need for medical students to be taught more about the key issues of mental illness – especially in terms of:

(i) *its extent:* the fact that one third of GP patients have psychosocial problems; one third of hospital outpatients are depressed; and one half or more of general medical in-patients are depressed[18];

(ii) *its impact* on all aspects of daily life – particulary marital problems, problems to children, sickness absence, and accidents.

(ii) *the major benefits gained from the early detection and treatment* of these disorders in primary care settings.

(iv) *the association between physical and psychological illness:*

(a) A strong primary association exists[23]. Doctors must realise that psychologically-ill patients are more likely to have a physical illness than are their psychologically well peers. *The physical health of many mentally-ill people is neglected*, and it is salutary to realise that the standardised mortality ratios of people discharged from psychiatric hospitals are grossly elevated by factors of 4 or 5 for cardiovascular disease, respiratory disease and malignancy – not just for deaths from suicide, accidents or violence[24].

(b) *Secondary associations* are perhaps more obvious: physical illness such as rheumatoid arthritis can cause psychological illness – including depression; and conversely, psychological illness – including depression – can be associated with physical illness; eg, chest infections caused by malnutrition and self-neglect.

(v) *Multiaxial assessment.* Medical students should therefore be taught the principles of *multiaxial assessment*, namely that, in assessing patients, attention must be paid to the physical, psychological, social and personality factors which contribute to their overall health status. Problems can occur in any axis, and difficulties in one do not preclude difficulties in another. Much physical and psychological illness has been missed by doctors who pay exclusive attention to only one axis, instead of viewing their patients in a more holistic manner[25].

(vi) Multidisciplinary liaison. Finally, we need to ensure that medical students are taught to liaise and work with a wide band of health professionals, including social workers and psychologists, as well as nurses; and to recognise their vital role in detecting possible depression in their patients and providing appropriate care.

Conclusion

Depression and anxiety affect people of both sexes, of all ages and social classes. They are both avoidable and treatable, and early detection and appropriate management significantly improve the prognosis. People and populations at risk can be identified and early intervention initiated. Effective treatment involves multidisciplinary co-operation and involvement of the patients themselves. Education of key health professionals – particularly GPs, medical students and members of the primary care team – is essential, not only about depression and anxiety in particular and mental health in general, but also about the close association between physical and mental illness, and the need for detection and management programmes to take account of, and be able to deal with, this association.

References

1. Office of Population and Censuses and Surveys. *Morbidity Statistics from General Practice – Third National Morbidity Survey 1981–2* London: HMSO, 1987

2. World Health Organisation. *Prevention of Mental, Neurological and Psychosocial Disorders.* Geneva: WHO, 1986

3. Caplan G. *Principles of Preventive Psychiatry* New York: Basic Books, 1964

4. Wing J K. *Rehabilitation and management of schizophrenia* In Handbook of Psychiatry Vol 3, Psychoses of Uncertain Aetiology (ed J K Wing and L Wing) Cambridge: Cambridge University Press, 1982

5. Jancar J. Consequences of longer life for the mentally handicapped *Geriatric Medicine* 1988, 18, 81–87

6. Goldberg D P, Creed F, Benjamin S. *Psychiatry in Medical Practice* London: Tavistock, 1987

7. Health Education. *Curriculum Guidance:* National Curriculum Council York 1990

8. Cutting J. *The Psychology of Schizophrenia* Edinburgh: Churchill Livingstone, 1985

9. Der G, Gupta S and Murray R M. Is Schizophrenia disappearing? *Lancet,* 1990, 335, 513–516

10. Rutter M L. Prevention of children's psychosocial disorders: myth and substance *Paediatrics* 1982, 70, no 6, 883–894

11. Office of Population and Censuses and Surveys. *Mortality Statistics: accidents and incidence 1988* HMSO DH4 no 14, 1990

12. Cobb S. Social support as a moderator of life stress *Psychosomatic Medicine* 1976, 38, 300–314

13. Henderson S, Byme D G, Duncan Jones P, Scott R, Alcock S. Social Relationships, adversity and neurosis: a study of associations in a general population sample *BrJ Psychiatry* 1980, 136, 574–583

14. Kessler R C and McLeod J. *Social Support and psychological distress in community surveys*. In Cohen S and Syme L (eds) Social Support and Health New York: Academic Press, 1984

15. Raphael B. Prevention intervention with the recently bereaved *Arch Gen Psychiatry* 1977, 34, 1450–1454

16. Gore S. The effect of social support in moderating the health consequences of unemployment
J Health Soc Behav 1978, 19, 157–165

17. Rutter M L, Madge N. *Cycles of Disadvantage* London: Heinemann, 1976

18. Goldberg D P, Huxley P. *Mental illness in the community: the pathway to psychiatric care* London: Tavistock, 1980

19. Department of Health and Social Security. *On the state of the public health: The Annual Report of the Chief Medical* Officer of the Department of Health and Social Security. London: HMSO, 1988

20. Johnson A L. Clinical trials in psychiatry *Psychol Med* 1983, 13, 1–8

21. Corney R, Murray J. *The evaluation of social interventions* In: The Scope of Epidemiological Psychiatry Edited by P Williams, G Wilkinson and K Rawnsley London: Routledge, 1989

22. Johnstone A, Goldberg D. Psychiatric screening in general practice Lancet, 1976, i, 605–608

23. Eastwood R. *The relationship between physical and psychological morbidity* In: The Scope of Epidemiological Psychiatry Edited by P Williams, G Wilkinson and K Rawnsley London: Routledge, 1989

24. Fox A J, Goldblatt P O. *Longitudinal Study – Sociodemographic Mortality Differences L S No 1 1971–1975* London: HMSO, 1982

25. Jenkins R, Smeeton N, Shepherd M. The classification of psychosocial problems in primary care *Psychological Medicine Monograph Supplement No 12* pp 1–59 Cambridge University Press, 1988

Further reading

1. Cohen S, Syme S L. *Social Support and Health* London: Academic Press, 1985
2. Duck S, Silver R C. *Personal Relationships and Social Support* London: Sage, 1990
3. Scottish Consultative Council on the Curriculum. *Promoting Good Health: Proposals for Action in Schools* Scottish Health Education Group: Edinburgh 1990

Address for contact

Dr Rachel Jenkins, Principal Medical Officer, Mental Health, Elderly and Disability Division, Department of Health, Room 303, Wellington House, London SE1 8UG.

3 Life Events and Social Support: Possibilities for Primary Prevention

GEORGE W BROWN, Professor of Sociology,
University of London

SUMMARY

Social factors play a central role in the aetiology of depression. Research on female samples indicates a number of promising avenues for preventive approaches. It is now possible to identify with reasonable accuracy those at high risk of depression. They are those with both internal risk factors (eg low self-esteem or on-going low level depressive or anxiety symptoms) and external risk factors (eg a negative interaction with partner or ongoing household difficulty). Opportunities for preventive action are argued to be most appropriate at 3 points in the life stage:

(i) In mid to late teenage years to correct adverse experiences in childhood.
(ii) At key transitional stages such as following divorce, or pregnancy outside a stable relationship.
(iii) Among vulnerable women at imminent risk of onset of depression.

In addition, intervention to stop episodes becoming chronic is recommended by means such as befriending to increase social support and the creation of positive events – changes such as rehousing or finding employment – and thus promote a 'fresh start'. There are a number of implications for professional practice arising from the research.

Introduction

My interest in the subject of depression is as a research worker and in this paper I see my purpose as providing some research insights into social factors which play a role in bringing about a depressive disorder or affect its course. I will focus on depression as there has been far more research on the role of social factors, although evidence begins to emerge that they may also play a significant role in related disorders such as anxiety[1,2,3].

Depression is particularly common in our inner cities. In any one year in areas such as Camberwell or Islington the prevalence of clinical depression (ie disorder assessed as roughly comparable to the severity seen in outpatients attending psychiatric clinics) is between 10 and 15 per cent of the female population. Added to this, at any one time half of the depressive conditions will have lasted for at least one year. This high rate of chronicity and the frequency with which people experience relapse represents a major public health problem.

Research over the past 20 years has shown that both the onset and course of depression can be powerfully influenced by psychosocial factors. There are, of course, biological concomitants, and research points to the intricate link between biological and psychosocial processes in most psychiatric disorders. With the development of knowledge about neurochemical and neuro-endocrine mechanisms and their link with pharmacological treatments, concern with biological aspects of disorders has greatly increased and the sheer bulk of such work has tended to swamp that concerned with psychosocial aspects. Therefore, while I do not wish to polarise issues of onset and course in terms of 'biology' versus 'psychosocial', it is of some importance to underline the significance of the latter – not least when discussing possible preventive implications of recent research.

Rates of 'caseness' of depression can be reliably measured and compared, and interesting results to emerge from various studies include:

(i) International studies of urban populations on the whole report rates of 'caseness' of depression not greatly different from those samples found in such centres in the United Kingdom. However, studies done within particular national populations show wide variations in prevalence: for example, middle-class women are less vulnerable to depression than working-class women, at least in the United Kingdom.

(ii) It has been consistently found, that fewer men than women develop depression. (However, differences might not in practice be quite as large as reported as men are typically more difficult to contact in general population enquiries and recognition might be made more difficult by the greater frequency of comorbid conditions such as alcoholism).

(iii) Some populations have exceptionally low rates of depression (eg, a non-inner city urban sample in Holland[4], and a rural district in the Basque Region of Spain[5]). It is also conceivable that populations exist where the overall rate of depression among women considerably exceeds that found in studies so far reported.

(iv) Factors associated with high rates of depression in one country – for example, for women in the United Kingdom, living with young children[6] might have little or no such effect in others (eg, in Spain[5] and Italy[7]). Such variations probably reflect the effect of cultural differences: the apparent failure of children at home to be a risk factor in some settings may well reflect differences in arrangements in the care of young children, and the value placed on the role of the mother.

A psychosocial model of depression

Our earliest studies in Camberwell[6] confirmed the basic picture emerging from insights provided by many research workers and practitioners – that most people get depressed because of some provoking event of a social nature, but that in the face of such events, some people are more vulnerable to clinical depression than others. Events which precede the majority of onsets of depression are severely threatening and are largely concerned with experiences of loss or rejection, disappointment or failure. But vulnerability to depression in the presence of such events is linked to factors such as social support, low self-esteem, and childhood experiences of parental indifference or neglect, and physical or sexual abuse[6,8].

The Islington Study

In 1980, my colleagues and I undertook a longitudinal study involving 400 women living in Islington, an inner-city area of London. We wanted to:

(i) further clarify psychosocial causes of acute depression;
(ii) determine factors responsible for the chronic course taken by some depressive disorders (some fifth of all episodes, at least in urban samples), and
(iii) identify possible areas for preventive intervention.

The population of women sampled was selected as likely to be at high risk for depression. They included either working-class mothers with a child living at home, or single parents from any social class. The study of acute onset was based on the 303 with no clinical depression at the time of the first interview. Of these women 32 (10.6 per cent) developed depression during the follow-up year, and 8 (25 per cent) of these became chronic – ie the symptoms of 'caseness' lasted 12 months or more. (As already noted the women were selected because they were likely to be somewhat more at risk than women in general and a somewhat lower onset rate would be expected among a random sample of women in an urban area).

Results from this study enabled us to produce the schematic causal model of clinical depression shown in Figure 3.1. This figure also indicates how effective prevention strategies might be planned to reduce both acute onset and chronic depressive illness. However, the relative simplicity of the diagram should not disguise the difficulties associated with prevention. Prevention, of course, is not only a matter of organising services and providing resources: it also requires social arrangements capable of sustaining and supporting preventive activities over the long term[9].

Onset of depression: the crisis situation

Among the 303 Islington women at risk for depression, 130 experienced a severe event in the follow-up year. Twenty nine of these 130 women became clinically depressed, showing that most women cope with such events without becoming depressed. However, of the 32 women who became depressed, 29 were women who experienced a severe event, showing that most depressions are preceded by a severe event. For just over a third of the 29 women with both a severe event and onset, the crisis presented a threat to their identity as a wife or mother about which very little could be done – at least in the immediate future. For most it was part of a long history of failure and disappointment in one or both of these roles. A second set, just under the size of the first, had a more diverse set of experiences. What they had in common appeared to be a

Figure 3.1 *Schematic causal model of clinical depression*

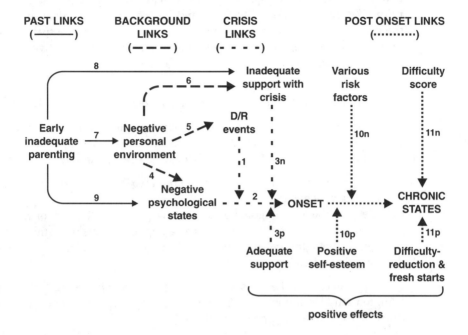

sense of imprisonment in a nonrewarding and deprived setting, with the event itself underlining how little they could do about extracting themselves. Any way forward appeared to be blocked. Events concerning poor housing, or debt, or both, were particularly common. A third set of women lost a core person they had known for some time. Most of these crises continue the same theme of failure or disappointment, loss or rejection. Overall, there was not much doubt about the conclusion to be drawn: the events presented for the most part, an integral threat to core aspects of the sense of identity and self-worth of the women[11].

Difficulty (D) and role conflict (R) events (link 1, figure 3.1)

Some severe events were much more likely to provoke depression than others. Severe events which matched an ongoing marked difficulty were one example – for instance, the difficulty of a single mother whose son had left home after a quarrel and who for some time since had refused to talk to her, being 'matched' by the event of learning he had been sent to prison. Most of the matching difficulties (ie, matching D-events) had been present for more than a year.

Severe events which match a prior role confict (R-events) have a similar effect; and among the Islington women conflicts between work and domestic responsibilities were particularly common. For example, one mother's concern (detected at the first interview) about coping with both work demands and the care of her 12 year old daughter were matched when her child was caught stealing from her. The occurrence of either a D-event or R-event increased risk of depression threefold when compared with other severe events[11]. Just over half the 32 Islington women who became depressed had experienced such a prior D/R event. As both difficulties and role conflict can be detected before the occurrence of a matching event some possiblity for preventive action is indicated, although, as will be seen, there may be more effective ways of identifying high risk women.

Support in crisis situations (links 3n and 3p in figure 3.1)

However, severe events, even when matching, did not inevitably lead to depression. Much appeared to depend on the effectiveness of support with the event. Effective 'crisis support' was defined by three criteria:

(i) The presence of someone close in whom the person 'at risk' may confide about the severe event.
(ii) Receipt of active, ongoing emotional support from that person.
(iii) The avoidance, by the person giving support, of making any negative comments about the person seeking help (ie to him or herself personally) during the required period of support.

The apparent crucial effect of such crisis support is clearly demonstrated in the Islington study, although the findings need to be replicated and ultimately tested in experimental type research.

In order to simplify, Table 3.1 deals only with the support received by married women from a husband or partner. It shows that:

- Married women who at first interview said they were able to confide in their husbands, and who received support from him (as defined above) when a severe event occurred were unlikely to get depressed (4 per cent only).
- Those who did not confide in their husbands at the time of the first interview, and did not receive crisis support either, were, as expected, at high risk of depression (26 per cent).
- Women were particularly at high-risk if they were confiding in their husband at the earlier point, but did not receive the crisis support they were expecting, ie they were 'let down'.

Table 3.1 *Confiding in husband at first interview, crisis support during the follow-up year and onset of depression among those with a provoking agent (86 married Islington women)*

Confiding in husband at first interview	Crisis support from husband during follow-up		
	YES	NO	TOTAL
	% onset	% onset	% onset
YES	4 (1/28)	37 (7/19) 'let down'	17 (8/47)
NO	25 (2/8)	26 (10/38)	24 (12/50)

(Crisis support not known for 3)

Further results, not shown in Table 3.1 provided additional insights. Among the 42 married women who neither expected nor received crisis support from their husbands, 18 received adequate support from someone else named earlier as 'very close' (usually a woman), and only one of these became depressed (link 3p, figure 3.1). And nearly all single mothers who were confiding in someone seen as very close at first contact, received support in subsequent crises. Thus the risk of depression in single mothers was more to do with lacking support in the first place, while for married women it was often to do with being 'let down'.

These findings highlight the importance of the quality of core relationships in the genesis of depression. For married women, the quality of the marital relationship, and for single mothers, their degree of social isolation might usefully be examined when first assessing the risk of acute onset depression[8,12].

Also related to risk of subsequent depression was whether or not the women, when seen at the first interview, had either low self-esteem or chronic sub-clinical symptoms of depression or anxiety. However, such negative psychological factors (ie internal risk factors) were usually not sufficient on their own to produce depression. External risk factors, in the form of a D/R event (link 1, figure 3.1) or inadequate personal support during a crisis situation involving a severe event (link 3) were usually also necessary. *Internal and external risk factors combined* were associated with a particularly high risk. This result has preventive implications because, as it turns out, both components can be recognised *before* any onset. The psychological factors were, as already conveyed, measured at the time of first contact. And the external factors occurring in the follow-up year (D/R event or inadequate support) were predicted at the time of first interview by a simple index. This involved taking account of either negative interaction with husband (or social isolation for single mothers) or negative interaction with a child at home. The combination of internal and external risk factors could therefore be identified at the time of first contact (ie before any depression). In Islington only 23 per cent of women (without clinical depression) were considered at high risk in these terms, and 75 per cent of all onsets of depressive disorder (24/32) recorded in the follow-up year occurred among this relatively small group of women. It may be possible to identify a small group of high risk women by taking account of low self-esteem, chronic sub-clinical symptoms of anxiety or depression and certain shortcomings in core relationships. The study therefore implies certain courses of action for prevention once women at high risk for an imminent onset within the next 12 months have been identified:

1. to work on changing the vulnerability factors eg through use of cognitive therapy to reduce negative interaction with partner or child;
2. to reduce ongoing difficulties likely to lead to future matching difficulty or role conflict events eg by social work contact;
3. to increase social support eg by befriending and thus increase chances of being supported once a severe event occurs.

Since such women have high attendance at GPs' surgeries (either for their own complaints or their children's) targeting them in surgeries for preventive action with the GP's support would seem the most practical.

Poor parenting and its relation to depression

Lack of adequate care in early childhood (involving marked parental indifference, physical and sexual abuse) is also associated with a high risk of depression in adulthood. Early studies suggested that events such as a child's loss of mother before 11 years-of-age were significant predisposing factors. More recent research indicates that the *effects* of the loss in terms of quality of parental care rather than the loss itself are more important[13,14]. For example, poor quality replacement parental care can lead to rejection, neglect and physical or sexual abuse of the child. Girls exposed to such experiences before 17 irrespective of whether or not it is associated with loss of mother have double the rate of low self-esteem as adults[15] (see link 7, Figure 3.1) and such links in turn increase risk of depression. As a rough estimate the rate of depression in inner-city areas would be reduced by at least a third if damaging early experiences related to poor parenting or sexual abuse could be prevented or their presence predicted, recognised and addressed more effectively.

These findings therefore have potentially important implications for prevention strategies. For example, befriending schemes such as Newpin in Southwark, and Home-Start (see Chapter 13) address the acknowledged link between depression in mothers, and child abuse and neglect. Other possible key points for intervention later in life include those associated with the early recognition of problems associated with the choice of an unsupportive, 'undependable' male partner, pre-marital pregnancy, and housing or employment.

The challenge of chronic depression

Why do acute episodes become chronic?

As already noted a quarter of the depression which developed in the Islington women lasted at least one year. In the light of other research carried out in urban settings this proportion was expected. One of the major research questions to be answered is thus, 'Why do acute episodes of depression become chronic?' (link 10). Ongoing marked difficulties relate to such chronicity and might well help to perpetuate a depressive disorder[6]. Another clue to what is going on lies in the finding that depression among Islington women was less likely to become chronic among those who had high self-esteem (based on positive comments that the woman made about herself at the time of the first interview). Such comments predicted the length of depressive episode among the 32 onset cases in the Islington study, and even recovery among women already chronically depressed[16].

Improvement and recovery

Improvement and recovery often occurred among the Islington depressed women following a certain type of 'positive event' – as long as the episode had lasted at least 4 months. The events on occasions involved the actual resolution or reduction in the difficulties stemming from the severe event that provoked the depressive episode in the first place. Such 'positive' changes could be characterised by, for example:

(i) reduction in ongoing difficulties (eg, improved housing conditions, marital discord, and ongoing family problems)
or
(ii) a fresh-start event – ie, something which (although it might be quite unpleasant) suggests hope of improvement in terms of an ongoing difficulty or deprivation. One influential view of depression is that it is often essentially about hope or to be more specific, lack of it – and hope is often a scarce commodity in inner-city populations. For the Islington women, examples of fresh-start events included: reconciliation with an estranged son and daughter-in-law after the birth of a second grandchild; starting divorce proceedings against a violent husband; a woman finding a job which relieved considerable financial difficulties and tension at home; and an extremely violent husband being jailed for several years because of his murderous attack on the woman and her mother.

There were exceptions, although approaching two-thirds of women recovering or improving had one such positive event or change. The most common group of exceptions were a small group who had become depressed after a bereavement (loss of a child or husband). For people like these, it seems likely that time and appropriate support will be the most important factors associated with recovery.

Adverse effects of depression on dependant children

Chronic depression causes significant suffering for individuals and has adverse immediate and long-term effects on their dependant children, close family and associates. For example, higher rates of accidents in children of depressed mothers have been reported[17].

The adverse effects on dependant children and the possibilities for prevention were highlighted by a follow-up survey of the Islington women who became depressed and their daughters (by then aged 15–24) eight years after the initial study[18]. Psychiatric disorders at 'case' level – including depression, anxiety and eating disorders – were found in approximately nine per cent of the daughters. Several already had babies – many of them as single mothers. Their problems were related to a history of chronic or episodic depression in the mother and even more closely, to inadequate parenting. These findings underline the value of any intervention capable of preventing such adverse long-term 'generational' effects.

Lifespan monitoring: periods of transition

Such findings make it increasingly clear that research needs to study women (and men also) over their lifespan. Some people will be found to suffer a brief episode of depression, say lasting 5 to 6 weeks and never have another. For others, depression will recur, or will last for several years. To study these differences, new concepts are needed, and we have recently been developing a notion of periods of transition, ie, times in a person's life when their vulnerability is most exposed, and they are least protected by usual structures and relationships. Decisions and commitments can be made at points of transition that may affect vulnerability for years to come, such as when moving from the parental home to marriage; from a children's home to adult responsibility; from a violent marriage to living alone.

For women, one of the risks at such a transition period relates to forming a partnership with an 'undependable' man. A man may be judged 'undependable' in the sense of factors such as infidelity, unpredictable provision of money for housekeeping, violence or poor living arrangements and such men probably play a central role in a good deal of long-term depression. These unhappy relationships are difficult to explain or study, but they probably reflect a subtle mixture of personality factors, structural environmental influences and basic biological responses. Take for example (albeit a somewhat extreme one) the following.

Case study

A woman in our survey had had a history of sexual abuse and lack of care – her father had tried on several occasions to strangle her mother. She escaped to a homeless persons' hostel and met there a man with a similarly deprived background.

The couple lived together happily for the first two years. She got pregnant and gave birth to twins, her partner then started to become violent and this continued for several years – until she left. Within a few weeks she was living with another man and he was violent from the very start. When first seen by us, her problems had lasted 10 years and she had been depressed for most of that time.

Many factors probably contributed to this woman's repetition of so unfortunate a choice of partner – for example, the fact of living in the same homeless person's hostel, sharing of early unhappy experiences, the fact that by the time of her marriage break-up, the woman's self-esteem was very low and she could not believe anyone could want her, that she could not bear to be left alone. Thus it becomes easier to at least suspect why she leapt into such an unsatisfactory relationship again the second time around. Structural environmental and personality factors undoubtedly infuence choices made at such transition periods. Of course, there may also be a great deal of luck involved too. It is, of course, very much an open question how far choices could be influenced in such situations.

Conclusion

Much of the depression seen in medical as well as in psychiatric practice is the immediate result of problems of living. It follows that our general way of life and cultural practices as a whole need to come under scrutiny – not necessarily always to change them in any straight forward sense, but at a minimum to provide more effective support and guidance. General practice, education and employment come readily to mind as means of providing additional support. Any study of the management of depression must encourage non-medical as well as medical input and collaboration.

Psychiatrists should give a lead and, for example, think more in terms of education, motivation, delegation and example. Such actions would influence a wider group of people and encourage prevention initiatives locally. GPs, health visitors and the police could learn more about the links between life events, support and depression. They would then be better able to recognise the vulnerability of their client groups and offer more constructive support. With the back up of psychiatrists, or primary care workers, communities could strengthen existing, or set up new voluntary support projects such as befriending schemes. All these and similar proposals require attention to training (as also indicated by other authors in this book). However, given suitable professional guidance, such services can provide ongoing, effective support and, I believe, significantly decrease both acute onset and chronic depression. Once such general services are in place it would be easier to assess the need for specialist services based on more traditional therapeutic lines.

References

1. Barlow D H. *Anxiety and its disorders*. New York: Guilford Press, 1988

2. Brown G W, Lemyre L, Bifulco A. Social factors and recovery from anxiety and depressive disorders: a test of specificity. *Br. J Psychiatry* (in press) 1992.

3. Brown G W, Harris T O, Eales M J. Early life experiences and anxiety and depressive disorders in an inner-city population: issues of aetiology and comorbidity. 1992 (manuscript)

4. Hodiamont P G, Het Zoeken van Zieke Zielen, Nijmegan Instituut sociale Geneekunde, 1986

5. Gaminde I, Uria M. Desordenes affectivos u factores sociales en la comunidad, 1988

6. Brown G W, Harris T O. *Social Origins of Depression: A Study of Psychiatric Disorder in Women*. London: Tavistock, 1978

7. Lora A, Fava E. Provoking agents, vulnerability factors and depression in an Italian setting: a replication of Brown and Harris' model. *Journal of Affective Disorders*, 1992 (in press)

8. Brown G W, Bifulco A, Andrews B. Self-esteem and depression: 3. Aetiological issues. *Social Psychiatry & Psychiatric Epidemiology*. 1990, 25, 235–243.

9. Brown G W. A psychosocial view of depression. In: D H Bennett & H Freeman (Eds) *Community Psychiatry*; Churchill-Livingstone 1991.

10. Brown G W. Life events and meaurement. In: G W Brown and T O Harris (Eds) *Life Events and Illness* London: Unwin & Hyman, 1989

11. Brown G W, Bifulco A, Harris, T O. Life events, vulnerability and onset of depression: some refinements. *British Journal of Psychiatry*. 1987, 150, 30–42.

12. Brown G W, Andrews B, Harris T O, Adler Z, Bridge L. Social support, self-esteem and depression. *Psychological Medicine*. 1986, 16, 813–831.

13. Harris T O, Brown G W, Bifulco A. Loss of parent in childhood and adult psychiatric disorder: The Walthamstow Study 1. The role of lack of adequate parental care. *Psychological Medicine*. 1986, *16*, 641–659.

14. Bifulco A, Brown G W, Harris T O. Childhood loss of parent and adult psychiatric disorder: the Islington Study. *Journal of Affective Disorders*. 1987, *12*, 115–128.

15. Brown G W, Bifulco A, Veiel H, Andrews B. Self-esteem and depression: 2. Social correlates of self-esteem. *Social Psychiatry & Psychiatric Epidemiology*. 1990, *25*, 225–234.

16. Brown G W, Bifulco A, Andrews B. Self-esteem and depression: 4. Effect on course and recovery. *Social Psychiatry & Psychiatric Epidemiology*. 1990, 25, 244–249.

17. Brown G W, Davidson S. Social class, psychiatric disorder of mother, and accidents to children. *Lancet* 1978, 1: 378–387.

18. Andrews B, Brown G W, Creasey L. Intergenerational links between psychiatric disorder in mothers and daughters: the role of parenting experiences. *Journal of Child Psychology and Psychiatry*. 1990, *31*, 1115–1129.

Further reading

Brown G W, Harris T O. *Social Origins of Depression* London: Routledge, 1978

Brown G W, Harris T O. *Life Events and Illness* London: Unwin and Hyman, 1989

Brown G W, Bifulco A, Andrews B. Self-esteem and depression 3 Aetiological Issues Social Psychiatry and Psychiatric Epidemiology 1989, 25 235–243

Herbst K R, Paykel E S. *Depression An Integrative Approach* Oxford: Heinemann Medical Books, 1989

Newton J. *Preventing Mental Illness* London: Routledge, 1988

Goldberg D, Huxley P. *Common Mental Disorders* London: Routledge, 1992

Address for contact

Professor George W Brown, Department of Social Policy and Social Science, Royal Holloway and Bedford New College, (University of London), 11 Bedford Square, London WC1B 3RA

4 Early Diagnosis and Secondary Prevention

DAVID GOLDBERG, Professor of Psychiatry,
University of Manchester

SUMMARY

Factors which determine the ability to detect depressive illness are known and can be modified by training. Doctors adept at detecting depression have a generally superior style of communication. They also manage the depression well and these skills are evident in their contact with other patients seen in day-to-day family practice. Failure to detect many cases of depression is a collusive phenomenon which involves doctor and patient. Evidence strongly indicates that early detection benefits patients. To facilitate this, more non-medical and 'lay' workers should be trained to help, especially with high-risk groups such as those with cancer, women after childbirth who have had a previous depressive illness, or the wives of prisoners.

Psychiatrists and prevention

In their daily clinical work, psychiatrists make only a modest contribution to the prevention of depression, since they provide second opinions on cases of depression that have not responded to treatment from the family doctor, and thus contribute to the tertiary prevention of the illness.

George Brown[1] (1990) has argued that psychiatrists have an important public health task to play in terms of delegation, education and example. Much of the routine care of depressive illness can be delegated to other health workers such as social workers and community psychiatric nurses, while the psychiatrist has an important educational role to play in providing medical students with their concepts of depressive illness, and in providing refresher courses and supervised training experiences to doctors, after they have qualified, in the recognition and medical management of depressive illness. These last functions will be discussed more fully in the remainder of this chapter.

The recognition of anxiety and depression in general medical practice

Anthony Mann (see Chapter 1) referred to our work on *hidden psychiatric morbidity*, a term which refers to cases of depression or anxiety which are confirmed by a psychiatrist at second stage interview, but which have been missed by the doctor in charge of the patient's treatment. Our earliest work[2] indicated that about one third of illnesses were missed when the GP was himself a qualified psychiatrist, but more recent studies have shown great variation between doctors in their ability to detect emotional distress among their patients. In Greater Manchester, for example, on average about 45 per cent of such illnesses are missed, while in London, the proportion is rather higher than this[3,4]. However, detection rates are very much higher if the patient included psychological symptoms among their presenting complaints: in this case about 95 per cent receive some sort of psychological diagnosis from their family doctor[5].

Failure to detect emotional distress as a collusive phenomenon

The patients whose psychological distress is not detected by their doctor are usually complaining of somatic symptoms, and may have real physical illnesses which do not account for their presenting symptoms. However, far from being unhappy with a doctor who has failed to detect emotional distress, both patient and doctor are typically satisfied with such consultations. Indeed, when one watches videotapes of consultations during which emotional distress is missed, one is struck by the *collusion* which occurs between patient and doctor to keep the consultation as 'non-psychological' as possible.

Patients are satisfied with such consultations for four main reasons:

(i) Doctors are usually courteous and kind to the patients, and this is naturally appreciated.
(ii) Doctors usually carry out a physical examination determined by the presenting symptoms. This reassures the patient that his or her complaints are being taken seriously, and the doctor, that nothing important has been missed.
(iii) When physical investigations are ordered, these reinforce the message that the somatic symptoms are being taken seriously, and satisfaction increases.
(iv) Symptomatic treatments – with analgesics, antacids or anti-inflammatory drugs – often provide relief for the patient. It is easier to take a medicine than to face up to distressing aspects of one's personal life, and both doctor and patient are relieved to resolve the problem without having to face personal difficulties.

Each step thus offers positive feedback and reinforces a mutual sense of achievement and satisfaction. The underlying depression remains undetected. Not surprisingly perhaps, doctors who miss depression usually do not know how to manage it. If they have not been taught to do this, why indeed bother to detect extra cases?

Interview behaviours and the ability to detect disorder

Behaviours which distinguish doctors good at detecting anxiety and depression from those who are not are listed in Table 4.1. *All* these behaviours may be taught and modified quite easily by training using video feedback of actual interviews between the doctor and his patients.

Patients interviewed by *doctors good at detecting distress* seem to make the task easier for the doctor[6]. They give more verbal cues, show more distress in their

Table 4.1 *Medical behaviours which distinguish doctors able to detect emotional distress among their clients, and which can be easily modified by training*

Start of the interview
  Makes eye contact with patient
  Is able to clarify complaint

General interview skills
  Picks up verbal cues
  Picks up non-verbal cues
  Can deal with over-talkativeness
  Deals with interruptions well
  Is not 'buried' in the notes

Types of question
  Asks directive 'psychiatric questions'
  Asks closed 'psychiatric questions'
  Makes supportive comments
  Asks about home

voice, and are more physically restless. Doctors who were good at detecting distress asked more directive psychiatric questions, were more likely to ask questions which followed directly on from what the patient had just said and were able to look things up in the notes without reducing the cues relating to distress emitted by the patient. In contrast, patients interviewed by *doctors poor at detecting distress* kept their voices under control, showed less emotion and kept their hands still. These doctors spent more time talking and were more likely to start giving the patient information in the first minute or two of the interview – perhaps as a prelude to terminating the interview.

Millar and Goldberg[7] have shown that doctors better able to detect disorder are also better able to manage it, and these differences hold up not only for patients with high scores on the psychological screening test, but for those with low scores as well. Whatever the patient's complaint, the doctor with better detection skills gives more information and advice to the patient, and gives them better information about any prescribed medication. They are therefore *better communicators* than those colleagues who habitually miss significant emotional distress among the patients consulting them.

Differences in interview behaviours are also evident when patients with high scores on the psychiatric screening test, the General Health Questionnaire (GHQ) are considered. Doctors who are good at detecting distress tend to ask a *directive social question* early in the interview – thus allowing themselves to leave the discussion of symptoms and to focus on personal matters. 'What is happening in the patient's life now?' Doctors who miss psychological disorders do not ask these questions; their definition of illness is much narrower.

Early detection. Benefit or not?

In 1976, Alan Johnstone, a family practitioner from Yorkshire, and I reported that a GP could decrease a patient's psychological distress by an average of 2.8 months if, at the first interview, he knew that the patient had a high score in the GHQ[8]. The National Institute of Mental Health (NIMH) in the USA followed up these findings in two substantial studies[9,10]. Neither confirmed our results, for two main reasons:

(i) The research was imposed upon the doctors, rather than something they wished to do themselves; thus many doctors did little with the information that they were given.

(ii) The doctors were merely told the GHQ score, rather than being given help in how to manage the additional information.

Other studies have been more supportive. Zung and her colleagues[11] randomised patients with high scores on a depression screening test and reassessed them four weeks later. In the index group, the physician was given the score and was free to decide whether or not to treat the patient. Of the group whose depression was detected and treated, 68 per cent had improved, compared with only 28 per cent of those detected but untreated, and 18 per cent in the undetected control group. Rucker and his colleagues[12] allowed physicians to re-interview patients if a depression screening score was high but they had missed the depression; this resulted in altered treatment plans for 20 per cent of the patients seen in the clinic. Rand and her colleagues[13] had the idea of randomising doctors rather than patients. The index residents were given training in how to deal with feedback of a high GHQ score, and in these doctors, GHQ feedback produced a two-fold increase in the number of psychiatric diagnoses and a significant increase in the prescription of antidepressants.

Two naturalistic studies have shown that depression detected by the family doctor has a better outcome than depression which is missed. Freeling and his colleagues[14] showed that undetected depression lasts longer than detected depression. Ormel and colleagues[15] confirmed this and showed that the better outcome in the detected group was not because they had received a particular treatment. Our original study in Yorkshire, and these recent findings suggest that improvement is often linked to the fact that personal distress has been shared with another person. Taken together, the results suggest that early detection of depression confers benefit on the patient.

Detection of depression in high risk groups

Jennifer Newton[16] and George Brown have emphasised the importance of targeting preventive strategies on high-risk groups. It is intuitively easy to see that it would be wasteful to devote resources to populations who are unlikely to get depressed. If we were to offer a preventive strategy to random samples of the population we would waste more than 90 per cent of our efforts. Holden, Sagovsky and Cox[17] have described successful preventive work with women who became depressed after childbirth, and Maguire and his colleagues[18] have shown that women who were depressed and received treatment following mastectomy were significantly less depressed than those whose depression was not detected. These results are still not conclusive. Linda Gask for example, has been unable to prove that interview training courses improved the detection of *severe* depression (see Chapter 5). A randomised controlled study of people with high GHQ scores on the medical wards of a district general hospital has also given a null result[19]. However, it is not easy to show an effect in this type of study because:

(i) Patients do not always receive the intervention the researchers hope for. People thought to have an illness may receive no specific treatment. In the general hospital medical wards, patients in Gater's study received the recommended treatment only until they were discharged. Poor communication between the hospital and family doctors meant that the latter remained unaware of the recommended treatment which, in most cases then ceased.

(ii) Severe depression is a fairly low-prevalence disorder. Any screening procedure therefore has a low positive predictive value.

(iii) All depressive illness has a fairly high spontaneous remission rate. About half the patients will have been ill for more than one year.

In 1974, Kincey, an MSc student at Manchester University,[20] offered counselling to a randomly selected sample of widows who had been prematurely bereaved, but was unable to show a significant benefit when they were compared with controls who had not been counselled. With hindsight, the correct strategy would have been to have offered treatment only to those women who were markedly depressed, and then to have ensured that those treated did in fact receive optimal treatment. It is to be hoped that such designs will be used by the next generation of investigators.

Conclusion

The factors which determine the ability to detect depressive illness are known, and can be modified by training. The ability to detect depression is part of a generally superior communicative style: doctors who are good at detection are also good at management. Failure to detect many cases of depressive illness is a collusive phenomenon affecting both doctor and patient. The available evidence favours the idea that early detection has some value. Finally more work should be done by 'lay' people and non-medical staff with high-risk groups.

References

1. Brown G. *Some public health aspects of depression*. In: Goldberg D, Tantam D, eds. The public health impact of mental disorder. Bern: Hogrefe and Huber, 1990.

2. Goldberg D, Blackwell B. Psychiatric illness in general practice. *BMJ* 1970;**2**:439–453.

3. Marks J, Goldberg D, Hillier V. Determinants of the ability of general practitoners to detect psychiatric illness. *Psychol Med* 1979;**9**:337–353.

4. Boardman A P. The General Health Questionnaire and the detection of emotional disorder by general practitioners: a replicated study. *Br J Psychiatry* 1987;**151**,373–381.

5. Goldberg D, Bridges K. Somatic presentations of psychiatric illness in the primary care setting. *J Psychosom Res* 1988;**32**:137–144.

6. Davenport S, Goldberg D, Millar T. How psychiatric disorders are missed during medical consultations. *Lancet* 1987;**ii**:439–441.

7. Millar T, Goldberg D. Determinants of the ability of general practitioners to manage common mental disorders. Med Educ 1991. (submitted)

8. Johnstone A, Goldberg D. Psychiatric screening in general practice: a controlled trial. *Lancet* 1976;**i**:605–608.

9. Hoeper E, Nycz G, Kessler L, Burke J, Pierce W. The usefulness of screening for mental illness. *Lancet* 1984;**i**:33–35.

10. Shapiro S, German P, Skinner E, et al. An experiment to change detection and management of mental morbidity in primary care. *Med Care* 1987;**25**:327–339.

11. Zung L, Magill M, Moore J. Recognition and treatment of depression in a family medicine practice. *J Clin Psychiatry* 1983;**4**:1–9.

12. Rucker L M, Frye E, Cygan R. Feasibility and usefulness of depression screening in medical out-patients. *Arch Intern Med* 1986;**146**:729–731.

13. Rand E, Badger L, Coggins D. Towards a resolution of contradictions: utility of feedback from the GHQ. *Gen Hosp Psychiatry* 1988;**10**:189–196.

14. Freeling P, Rao B, Paykel E, Sireling L, Burton R. Unrecognised depression in general practice. *BMJ* 1985;**290**:1880–1883.

15 Ormel H, Koester M, van den Brink W, van de Willige G. *The extent of non-recognition of mental health problems in primary care and its effect on management and outcome.* In: Goldberg D, Tantam D, eds. The public health impact of mental disorder. Bern: Hogrefe & Huber, 1990.

16. Newton J. *Preventing mental illness.* London: Routledge, 1988.

17. Holden J M, Sagovsky R, Cox J L. Counselling in general practice settings: a controlled study of health visitor intervention in the treatment of post-natal depression. *BMJ* 1989;**298**:223–226.

18. Maguire P, Tait A, Brooke M, Thomas C, Sellwood R. The effect of counselling upon psychiatric morbidity associated with mastectomy. *BMJ* 1980;**281**:1454–1456.

19. Gater R, Goldberg D, Evanson J, Lowson K, McGrath G, Tantam D, Million L. The detection and treatment of psychiatric illness in a general medical ward: a cost-utility analysis. J Psychosom Res 1991. (submitted).

20. Kincey V. The effects of bereavement counselling on prematurely bereaved widows. Manchester, England: University of Manchester, 1974. (unpublished MSc. thesis).

Further reading

Goldberg D, Huxley P. *Common mental disorders: a bio-social model.* London: Routledge, 1991.

Address for contact

Professor David Goldberg, University of Manchester, Department of Psychiatry, Withington Hospital, West Didsbury, Manchester, M20 8LR.

5 Teaching Psychiatric Interview Skills to General Practitioners

LINDA GASK, Senior Lecturer in Psychiatry,
Royal Preston Hospital

SUMMARY

Psychiatric interviewing skills can be improved by using video and audio feedback recordings of clinical consultations. Skills can be quickly and easily learned, and a problem-based approach which provides a useful model for teaching these skills is described in some detail. Teaching packages now exist to improve the detection and management of problems, such as alcohol misuse and 'somatisation'. Doctors should know how to detect patients' problems effectively and engage them in receiving appropriate help, even if they intend to refer them to specialist counselling.

Psychiatric interview skills: Are they really necessary?

The ability to establish and maintain effective communication links with patients, their families, and each other is a prime factor affecting the quality of care provided by GPs and members of primary health care teams. Acute physical distress and life-threatening conditions demand rapid diagnosis and skilled medical attention. Emotional concomitants may, at least initially, seem to be of secondary concern. Nonetheless, they may be addressed by routine crisis management procedures; by successful treatment of the problem itself; by counselling services contacted once the cirsis is over; and, outside the clinical setting, by the patient's personal and social support networks.

Most patients however, do not present their GPs with acute, life-threatening conditions. They need doctors who are good listeners; who can help them ventilate their feelings; bolster their confidence; differentiate physical from other problems. When the latter are emotional, very specific and delicate interventions are usually necessary. The doctor might need for example, to persuade a patient or his family, that the physical symptoms mask depression; that an anti-depressant, not a pain killer, will relieve the pain; that referral to a psychiatrist is a positive step, not a lethal blow to an already battered self-esteem.

The knowledge and skills required for this type of interaction are known and can be taught. The need for formal training must be recognised. A little knowledge acquired and applied somewhat haphazardly amid the competing interests and demands of a busy general practice is unlikely to benefit either doctor or patient. Nor does employment of a trained counsellor adequately compensate for lack of such skills in the GP and practice team. Doctors unable to detect emotional disorders or negotiate appropriate management programmes with their patients inevitably waste much valuable time and goodwill through wrong referrals. Such delays jeopardise the chances of a quick recovery.

Teaching psychiatric interview skills

Psychiatric interview skills suitable for use in general practice and primary care settings cannot be acquired passively via indirect association with specialist colleagues. For example, psychiatrically-trained professionals, may be theoretically members of a primary care team. But many still practice in isolation, seeing patients referred to them in rooms set apart for that purpose in the health centre. Skills and knowledge are best transferred and reinforced by active processes; by formal training; by regular participation in team planning and management programmes. Effective transfer has reciprocal benefits: the 'experts' gain insight into everyday aspects of general practice; team work and patient care are improved.

Two major movements have influenced the teaching of psychiatric interview skills in general practice:

Non-directive counselling

This technique, learned by many GP vocational trainees, is based on an hour-long interview. Standard GP appointments last only 10 minutes. Its validity in such settings is thus being challenged. Nancy Rowland and her colleagues at York have even suggested that GPs should not do counselling[1]. This radical proposal seems to question the valuable contributions made by 'Balint'-trained GPs and for others, the opportunity to pursue an important interest.

Video feedback

The use of video feedback to improve interview skills was first described and researched with medical students in 1978 by Peter Maguire and his colleagues in Manchester[2]. David Pendleton and Theo Schofield in Oxford[3] have also done much to demystify the procedure for GPs. In Canada, Art Lesser[4] has developed techniques in group teaching which have greatly influenced my own work, including that funded since 1985 in Manchester, by Research and Development for Psychiatry (RDP).

The technique for giving video or audio feedback is quite straightforward. GPs record their own clinical consultations on audio or, preferably, video tape and play these back in the company of colleagues assisted by a trained group facilitator. One-to-one viewing with an experienced teacher is also possible. In the group teaching session, anyone may stop the tape, provided that they can then offer constructive criticism: ie, say what they would have done or said at that point in the consultation. This procedure protects the interviewer who, after the meeting can test the suggestions made in subsequent consultations. Stopping the tape allows new skills to be rehearsed within the group. Further videos may be similarly viewed to assess progress or address specific problems.

The problem-based interview: providing structure

The problem-based interview, unlike conventional psychiatric or medical history-taking concentrates on the exploration and clarification of the patients' presenting problems – rather than simply arriving at the 'diagnosis' which might not always be particularly useful, where anxiety and depression in primary care are concerned, in predicting outcome or indicating appropriate interventions. It is the model used in video feedback sessions to teach the early detection and effective management of emotional disorders in general practice. The GP learns to help patients discern and clarify their problems, to assess these accurately, and then, with the patient, to negotiate an appropriate and agreed course of management[5]. The four main steps involved in this process require:

(i)   Accuracy in sensing and detecting patients' problems.
(ii) Concise, complete description of elicited problems.
(iii) Determination of patients' motivation and ability to change.
(iv) A mutually-agreed plan for solving or improving the problems (based on information gained from (i)–(iii)).

Basic skills

Beginning the interview: sources of information

Three important sources of information immediately available from the interview are:

(i)   What the doctor hears (verbal content and vocal cues).
(ii) What the doctor sees (non-verbal and visual cues).
(iii) What the doctor feels (emotional (personal response) cues).

It is not only *what* the patient says but *how* it is said which matters. The *tone* of voice is very revealing. *Posture, general appearance* and *demeanour* all provide valuable clues. Doctors must also examine their *emotional responses* to patients. Do they feel sympathy, anger – dislike? If the last, is it possible that the patient has the same effect on people close to him or her in their daily lives? Have they, as a result, no-one-else with whom to share their problems – a key factor in depression (see Chapter 3)?

The doctor learns to pick up and use cues effectively; to use open-ended questions which give patients a better opportunity to express their own feelings, rather than respond to the clinician's assumptions or present only information which they believe would be accepted by him. The doctor asks patients to clarify points, asking for examples wherever possible; responding to and using non-verbal cues: 'I can see you're feeling quite upset at the moment. Would you like to tell me more about it?'. The patient's own perspective and opinions are made to matter – at a time when self-doubt might have whittled away confidence.

Demonstrating empathy enables the doctor to assure the patient (without necessarily reaching agreement over specifics) that the reason for consultation is valid. 'I can see this has really got you down. You must have a lot on your plate.' Letting the patient know that you understand how tough life can be, can open unexpected doors and speed up the recovery process.

Health beliefs and concerns influence the way patients perceive and present their problems. Simple questions such as, 'What do you think has been causing your pain?', or, 'Is there anything in particular *you've* been worried about?' again value the patient's opinion; help clarify or correct misconceptions. The doctor and patient continue working together.

Controlling the interview can prove difficult if a patient rambles. Doctors learn how to bring people back to the point politely, using skills which show they are indeed listening – not merely being impatient.

Management and assessment

Once the basic principles above are understood and to some degree mastered, more complex issues of management and assessment are introduced to the course. Doctors are encouraged to bring along examples of problems they are facing with particular patients. Table 5.1 gives an idea of the type of patient and complexity of problems suitable for discussion by the group.

Specific skills taught during this stage enable doctors to help patients ventilate their feelings; negotiate agreement on management pogrammes; and most important, link presenting physical symptoms with life events and underlying psychological problems ie the essential skills of *reattribution*. Basic problem-solving skills needed for the effective management of anxious patients, and techniques suitable for special interviews – eg, seeing a mother and daughter

Table 5.1 *Patients suitable for discussion at seminars teaching problem-based interview techniques*

Patients with:

1. Overt psychiatric illness but management unclear.

    For example:
    a. Depression unresponsive to treatment(s)
    b. Non-specific anxiety

2. Specific problems evident

    For example:
    a. Marital difficulties
    b. Family conflict

3. Covert psychiatric illness suspected

    For example:
    a. Frequent attenders with multiple symptoms
    b. 'Pain' patients (frequent pain, uncertain origin)

together – are also included. Setting appropriate limits can pose problems. Determining how much time is available for treatment, compared to how much it is believed might be needed; and accepting that someone has not the capacity to change, are two examples of limit-setting dealt with by assessment and management training.

Evaluation

What effects have these programmes had on GPs, their patients and emotional illness?

Teaching

Evaluation studies of GPs in Manchester who completed training showed that both trainees and experienced GPs improved their interview skills[6,7] and these skills persisted over time[8].

Ten experienced GPs who received two hours tuition per week for 18 weeks (mean age 43.3 years and mean years in practice, 14.6) showed a statistically-significant improvement in both the use of direct psycho-social questions and clarifying comments and ability to detect and develop main problems. Closed questions were used less frequently. Other improvements were noted – eg, requests for specific examples, evidence of empathy, and ability to pick up affect-laden comments – but were not statistically significant[6].

We have also recently demonstrated that video feedback techniques can be used successfully to teach GP trainees how to impart interview skills to their students[9]. This process is greatly improved if the teachers use taped examples of their own consultations.

Doctor response

Feedback from experienced GPs who completed training courses on problem-based interview techniques showed:

(i)   Increased confidence in managing psycho-social problems.
(ii) Structure provided by the problem-based model was helpful.
(iii) Increased awareness of covert psychological factors.
(iv) Increased awareness of patients' vocal/verbal cues.
(v)   Increased taping of personal interviews.
(vi) Encouragement of trainees to tape their own interviews.

Impact on patient care and patient response

A recently completed study which explored the impact of teaching on patient care, satisfaction and clinical outcome[10] found: trained doctors made more references in case notes to patients' psychological states and psycho-social problems than untrained doctors ($p < 0.05$); they more often discussed the side-effects of medication ($p < 0.005$); and reached better agreement with patients about the nature of their problems. As a result, patients felt their problems were better understood ($p < 0.05$).

However, there was no demonstrable effect of training on compliance with medication or other treatment regimens.

Both the PSE and the GHQ scores showed a significant difference between index and control groups – baseline/one month and baseline/six months (GHQ only) for anxious *and* depressed patients; ie, *patients who were both anxious and depressed did best*. This is an important finding because these people are often difficult to handle in conventional surgery settings and put a heavy burden on their families, employers and primary care services. Doctors trained in psychiatric interview techniques felt much more confident about coping with these patients.

New horizons: specific skills teaching packages

Primary care workers are involved in an increasing variety of difficult, emotionally-charged activities – eg, talking to couples and families, counselling for sexual problems, bereavement counselling, and coping with patients with terminal illness – including cancer and HIV/AIDS. As a result, teaching packages are being developed to address particular skills required. Studies done in Oxford have shown that GPs trained in problem-solving techniques manage anxious patients very effectively[11]. I am currently developing a teaching package for the early detection and management of alcoholism, and have been involved with another on HIV-counselling-skills for GPs.

Professor Goldberg, Art Lesser and I, working with many GPs in North-West England, have also collaborated on a combined demonstration video package which deals with the difficult but essential skill of re-attribution. Patients who learn to understand and accept the links between physical symptoms and psychological disorders and their mutual association with day-to-day events will make better and more rapid progress. The package addresses very specific skills needed for this task and its use by this method. Their impact on patient care has now to be proven[12].

Conclusion

Video feedback techniques which record actual doctor/patient consultations, based on the problem-based interview model, may be used to improve doctors' psychiatric interviewing skills and thus promote the early detection and efficient management of emotional disorders – particularly anxiety and depression. These interview skills must be actively learnt: by formal training and by participation in team work shared with trained colleagues. Employment of a trained counsellor in a general practice does not compensate for a lack of interview skills in other members of the team – particularly the doctor. The GP must know how to detect patients' emotional problems and engage them in receiving appropriate help. A wider variety of teaching packages which address specific problems met in primary care practice is now available; their use by professionals with a basic training in interview skills should enable the latter to address areas of particular concern and interest more effectively and more efficiently. It is hoped that the growth of these skills amongst primary care professionals will ultimately become self-generating.

References

1. Rowland N, Irving J Maynard A. Can general practitioners counsel? *J R Coll Gen Pract* 1989;**39**:118–120.
2. Maguire P, Roe P, Goldberg D et al. The value of feedback in teaching interviewing skills to medical students. *Psychol Med* 1978;**8**:695–704.
3. Pendleton D Schofield T, Tate P, Havelock P. *The consultation: an approach to learning and teaching*. Oxford: Oxford University Press, 1984.
4. Lesser A L. The psychiatrist and family medicine: a different training approach. *Med Educ* 1981;**15**:398–406.
5. Lesser A L. Problem based interviewing in general practice. *Med Educ* 1985;**19**:299–304.
6. Gask L, McGrath G, Goldberg D, Millar T. Improving the psychiatric skills of established general practitioners. *Med Educ* 1987;**21**:362–368.
7. Gask L, McGrath G, Goldberg D, Millar T. Improving the psychiatric skills of the general practice trainee: an evaluation of a group training course. *Med Educ* 1988;**22**:132–138.
8. Bowman F, Goldberg D, Millar T et al. Does training in psychiatric interviewing skills persist? 1991. (submitted for publication).
9. Gask L, Goldberg D, Boardman J et al. Can general practitioners be taught how to teach psychiatric skills?: an evaluation of group training. 1991. (submitted for publication).
10. Gask L, Goldberg D. The impact on patient care, clinical outcome and patient satisfaction of improving the psychiatric skills of general practitioners. 1991. (in preparation).
11. Gath D, Catalan J. The treatment of emotional disorders in general practice: psychological methods versus medication. *J Psychosom Res* 1986;**30**:381–386.
12. Goldberg D, Gask L, O'Dowd T. The treatment of somatisation: teaching the techniques of reattribution. *J Psychosom Res* 1989;**33**:689–695.

Further reading

Neighbour R. *The Inner Consulation*. Lancaster: MTP Press, 1987.

Tucker D, Boulton M, Olson C, Williams A. *Meetings between experts: an approach to sharing ideas in medical consultations*. London: Tavistock, 1985.

Address for contact

Dr Linda Gask, Senior Lecturer in Psychiatry, Avondale Unit, Royal Preston Hospital, PO Box 66, Sharoe Green Lane, Preston PR2 4HT.

6 The Computer will see you now: Meeting the Challenge of Hidden Psychiatric Morbidity in General Practice

ALASTAIR WRIGHT,
Royal College of General Practitioners

SUMMARY

Hidden psychiatric morbidity poses a major challenge to the general practitioner and primary care team. This paper describes encouraging improvements to the rate of detection of psychiatric disorder in general practice which can be achieved through the use of computers and psychiatric questionnaires. These approaches are also helpful in developing effective management protocols. The computer is well accepted by patients who see it as an adjunct to – not a replacement for – doctor/patient contact. Although it is too early to prove that these methods lead to improved patient care, further research seems warranted.

Background

One of the biggest problems I face as a general practitioner (GP) is the patient who persistently presents somatic complaints without any sign of physical disease. For example, the patient who is always tired. Many such patients have an important psychological component to their illness which, if difficult to define, can go unrecognised by both the patient and the doctor. *Possible reasons for non-diagnosis of psychiatric disorders* in general practice include:

(i) *Short appointments.*
With the average consultation time less than 10 minutes, the diagnostic process is normally spread over several consultations. This is not a poorer method of diagnosis – just one which is appropriate for current working conditions;

(ii) *Doctor factors – bias and accuracy.*
Some GPs are biased towards physical illness and so find physical explanations for most symptoms. Others, depending on their interests and experience, are less accurate in their diagnoses; and – very important,

(iii) *Somatisation*.
Patients with hidden emotional problems invariably begin the consultation by complaining of a physical symptom, although it may be quite clear that the basic problem is psychological. A frequent association with this syndrome is *fat files* – ie, medical records which contain many negative results, and often, letters from many different specialists, explaining what is *not* wrong with the patient! Such fat files annoy me: they represent both a misuse of scarce and perhaps, costly, investigative resources and the unmet needs of a type of patient who is often very distressed.

The following discussion explains how I, as a GP working in a busy general practice, am, with my partners, addressing the challenge of hidden psychiatric morbidity. I hope this personal account will help colleagues in similar areas of primary care.

Research in general practice: a GP's viewpoint

Research projects are not easy to organise amidst the hurly burly of everyday practice. *Two special problems are common*:

(i) GPs have little access to trained interviewers;
and
(ii) it is very difficult to process and analyse large amounts of data within the practice itself (ie, where it is best understood).

However, GPs also have *two special advantages*:

(i) special questionnaires, prepared and tested by psychiatrists (see below);
and
(ii) a limitless resource of patient goodwill.

These advantages may be effectively combined, by using a microcomputer, to tackle and solve problems of hidden morbidity. The success we have had is encouraging and explains the title of my paper.

The GPs' psychiatric workload

Two research methods which may be used to indicate the extent of the psychiatric load are:

An overview of the prevalence of different illness groups

Figure 6.1 provides an estimate of the *prevalence* of different illness groups seen in my own practice. It is a general 'snapshot'; one which includes chronic illness and various problems – eg, digestive disorders in men, and genito-urinary in women – which are often difficult to define in purely physical (or psychological) terms.

New cases: the incidence of psychiatric illness

Another way of examining the GP's psychiatric workload is to look at *new* patients presenting over a one-year period and to compare those who com-

Figure 6.1: *'Snapshot' of the prevalence of different illness groups seen in a general practice*

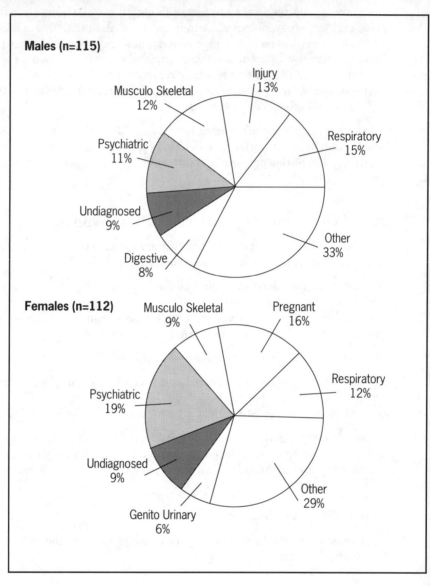

Figure 6.2 *One-year GP experience of new cases*

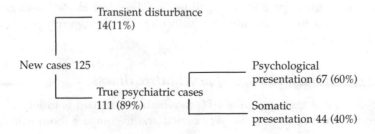

plain of somatic symptoms for which no physical explanation is found at the first consultation (*the somatic group*), with those who describe psychological problems (*the psychological group*). The results of these comparisons indicate the *incidence* of psychiatric illness in the practice (see Figure 6.2).

Conducting a research project in general practice

The project

A comparison of patients similar to the two groups described in 2 above, formed the basis of a study carried out in practice during 1988/1989, using microcomputers to help detect hidden psychiatric morbidity. A full report of this work appeared in the November 1990 issue of the *British Journal of General Practice*[1].

After a clinical assessment of a patient recruited to the study was completed and a provisional diagnosis reached, the research assistants invited each one (from both groups) to sit in front of the computer and, having shown each how to use the appropriate keys on the keyboard, left them alone, to answer a series of multiple-choice questions chosen from three reliable and well validated questionnaires – see below[2,3,4].

The results obtained were then used to assess each patient's psychiatric state and personality, and the social stresses and supports present in their daily lives. Using the computer in this way helped overcome the lack of an experienced interviewer and the frequent problem of unanswered questions found when paper questionnaires are used – (the computer required users to answer each question before the next one was offered).

Patient sample

Some 125 patients were recruited over the 12-month period – 91 women (aged 18 – 78 years, and 34 men (aged 21 – 64 years): 73 (58 per cent) presented *new* psychological problems (chronic 'cases' and psychotic patients were excluded), and 52 (42 per cent) had somatic symptoms for which no physical cause could be found. Both groups were equally likely to be assessed as 'cases' by a research psychiatrist.

Of the original 125, 14 (11 per cent) had only a transient disturbance: of the remaining 111 'true' psychiatric cases, 67 (60 per cent) presented psychological symptoms and 44 (40 per cent), somatic.

Patient response

Only two patients refused the invitation to take part in the study; none of the 125 who did so was unable to use the conventional keyboard or was worried by problems of confidentiality or 'impersonal' care. Indeed, they saw the computer as an adjunct to the traditional doctor/patient interview – ie, in much the same category as pathology and other laboratory tests or x-rays.

Participants commented favourably on: the thoroughness of the questions; the opportunity which using the computer gave them to clarify their thoughts about their problems (before their next appointment with the doctor); and pleasure associated with the interaction. *Their main reservation* was the ability to give only 'yes' or 'no' responses – many wanted to qualify their answers. At the six-month follow-up, 118 patients (94 per cent) completed the questionnaires. None refused. One patient in the psychological group had died, three had left the practice, and one was too ill to co-operate; two patients with somatic symptoms had also left.

Clinical diagnoses

(i)   *At recruitment*
Table 6.1 shows the initial diagnoses made on first contact.

Table 6.1:   *Clinical diagnosis at recruitment*

Patients			
Psychological group (N=73)		Somatic group (N=52)	
Diagnosis		Diagnosis	
Depression	38	Headache	13
Anxiety states (without depression)	27	Lassitude/anorexia	12
Alcohol problems	3	Other pains	7
Other	5	Giddiness	5
		Palpitations	3
		Other	12

There were no surprises. Patients presenting psychological problems received psychological diagnoses, and those offering somatic symptoms received a temporary *working* label which remained until psychiatric assessment was completed. Some of the presenting symptoms were quite odd: eg, twitching, 'restless legs'; itching skin (no physical cause); and breathlessness.

(ii)   *After six months*
Sixty-eight patients presented with psychological symptoms. The diagnosis was changed in only five – from anxiety to depression. Fifty patients from the somatic group were followed up, and of these, 13 received a psychiatric diagnosis in place of the 'working label' assigned at recruitment.

Determining quality care: Can the computer help?

The quality of patient care is easy enough to talk about; but in the reality of busy, changing and increasingly multi-faceted practice, consistently satisfactory standards are much more difficult to achieve *and* maintain. I agree with Rachel Jenkins' emphasis on the importance of looking at the whole patient – ie, at the physical, psychological and social aspects of their problems *together* (see Chapter 2). Table 6.2 shows how we used those terms of reference to determine patients' diagnoses and then to plan their care accordingly, in the belief that better quality care would follow.

Table 6.2: *Determining quality of care*

Status	Method used
Physical	Clinical examination (including laboratory test referral)
Psychological	A. Doctor's general assessment B. Psychiatric status (CIS) C. Personality (EPQ)
Social	Stresses and support (SPQ)

1. The physical examination is the easiest step – provided sufficient care is taken to match the clinical history with the signs found, and to clarify possible incongruities: if necessary by arranging appropriate referral and/or laboratory tests.

2. Psychological assessment requires skills and experience which, until recently, were generally considered to be outside the GPs' usual repertoire – even perhaps, outside their main area of responsibility.

(A) *The doctor's general (clinical) psychological assessment* involves interview techniques, personal insight and empathy (see Chapter 7), and the use of psychiatric questionnaires – ie, skills and resources which doctors can readily *learn, acquire* and *apply* in general practice. Referral to, and collaboration with, psychiatrist colleagues and relevant members of the secondary care and general practice teams also provide essential assistance, but I wish, here, to concentrate on the use of psychiatric questionnaires – and their delivery, where possible by computer.

(B) *Psychiatric status* is assessed mainly by two tests, the *28-item, General Health Questionnaire (GHQ)*[2], which is a pencil and paper test; and the *Clinical Interview Schedule (CIS)*[3]. The CIS is a semi-structured, standardised interview used by trained personnel and it thus agrees more closely with clinical judgement. A recently-produced computerised form – *The Interactive Psychosocial Assessment for Use in General Practice – Clinical Interview Schedule (IPSAG-CIS)*[4] – provides an easily-administered psychiatric review, suitable for use by GPs and trained members of the practice team. It gives an overall score for psychiatric status, lists the number of psychological and somatic symptoms experienced by the patient, and determines their severity. Psychiatrists can also use the CIS to establish reliable (and comparable) standards for 'case' identification. The questionnaire itself is rather difficult to administer without a computer.

The computer-compatible version of the GHQ is used as a comparison for the IPSAG computer interview. The final score gives an idea of the degree of psychiatric distress suffered.

(C) *Personality* is difficult to assess (score) by clinical interview alone. I adopted the paper-based *Eysenck Personality Questionnaire (EPQ)*[5] as it was well-reported in the literature and is not too difficult to use. Repeated use also helps: familiarity with administration and interpretation promotes greater confidence, and competence. To avoid possible patient overload at the initial session, and as personality is considered to be stable over time, the EPQ was completed at the six-month follow-up.

3. Social stresses and supports were measured by the *Social Problem Questionnaire (SPQ)* developed by Corney and Clare[6] which lists personal, social and marital status and the number of social problems.

Results

Tables 6.3 and 6.4 demonstrate the mean test scores of both groups, and differences in the symptoms described by each.

Table 6.3: *Mean test scores*

	Psychological Symptoms (Group 1)	Somatic Symptoms (Group 2)	Probability
Psychiatric state tests			
General Health Quest. '28'	16.8	12.6	<0.01
IPSAG computer interview	28.2	21.1	<0.01
Eysenck Personality Scores			
P score (tough mindedness)	2.6	1.8	<0.05
E Score (extraversion)	10.2	9.7	N.S.
N score (instability)	16.1	14.0	<0.05
Number of social problems	1.2	0.6	<0.01

(Psychiatric tests: *Both* groups equally likely to be thought 'cases' by a psychiatrist, but Group 1 more severe in terms of our definition of depression and anxiety states).

Table 6.4: *Individual symptoms: somatic compared to psychological patients*

The somatic group compared with the psychological group had:
  More severe
    Somatic symptoms
  Less severe
    Sleep disturbance
    Phobias
    Indecision
  Much less severe
    Irritability
    Depression
    Depressive thoughts
    Loss of concentration
    Anxiety
    Frequent checking
    Unwelcome thoughts
  No difference
    Tiredness
    Hypochondriasis
    Depersonalisation
    Derealisation

The psychiatric tests showed that both groups were equally likely to be considered 'cases' when judged by psychiatric criteria. The personality scores revealed that, although patients presenting psychological symptoms were surprisingly 'tough-minded', they were more unstable than their somatic counterparts, and experienced more severe degrees of anxiety and depression. This finding highlights the need to emphasise again that *computer tests do not remove the need for clinical assessment involving doctor/ patient interview – particularly when considering the risk of suicide*. Some patients seem to find it easier to express their suicidal thoughts to a computer than to a doctor: it is therefore essential to examine the questionnaires *very soon* after their completion – not after a weekend or holiday break!

Table 6.4 confirms what might have been predicted – that the somatic patients were not so irritable, or unable to concentrate, or as anxious or depressed as the psychological group – indeed their symptoms were less severe than those generally accepted for a diagnosis of classical depression or anxiety. However, no statistically-significant difference was found in the prognosis of each group: both were likely to have normal scores at the six-month review.

Potential of the computer

There is much more to psychiatric consultation than simple data collection. However, as noted above, the computer tests used in this general practice study were well-received by the patients. They were *not* seen as replacements for personal consultation, although they offered many a better chance to express and clarify their thoughts (including about suicide) than did the initial doctor/patient interview.

As a result of this response, we now offer computerised psycho-social testing as a practice service. It has proved useful in the detection, assessment and management of new patients' problems. Far from displacing clinical responsibility, the use of computers allows more time to analyse the patient's symptoms and reach better-informed decisions.

Discussion

As a result of our study, several issues needing further attention have been raised for discussion:

(i) *Somatisation*
Problems are usually more rapidly solved once their cause has been recognised. We need to know why so many people with psychosocial disorders present with somatic symptoms. Could it be that 'somatisation' represents a disorder in communication? If so, computers might help these patients express themselves more effectively.

(ii) *Measurement*
GPs aim to define patients' problems in physical, psychological and social terms. The means by which we can begin to *measure* these factors, and to improve our understanding of their individual and combined influences, are

being provided by the work of research psychiatrists and the advent of the desk-top computer.

(iii) *Prevention*

I believe that there are some areas of preventive work that can more readily be addressed by family doctors than others. For instance our role is crucial in helping to shorten the duration of illnesses (secondary prevention) and lessen the chance of chronic disability (tertiary prevention). Perhaps we can move towards primary prevention by giving earlier attention to physical symptoms which can be signs of stressful life circumstances. Perhaps cases of depression could be prevented in this way and suicide attempts also. About two thirds of the people who attempt suicide consult their GP within the month preceding the attempt. Surely there is scope for improvement there?

(iv) *Teamwork*

I am personally very committed to the team approach to health care. A few years ago, a consultant psychiatrist set up his clinic in our health centre. The advantages of this simple move have been multiple: he sees local patients at the centre, rather than at the hospital; GPs meet him on a regular basis; and we have begun to work more closely with community psychiatric nurses, psychologists and other professionals in mental health.

GPs are looking increasingly often to other health professionals for help with the recognition and care of patients with psychological problems. this multi-disciplinary co-operation, with its enormous pool of skills and resources, should lead to greatly-improved quality of care.

Modern technology has an important part to play. Data-gathering as described by Robert Gann (see chapter 12B), audio-visual teaching methods, personal tapes and cassettes on topics such as depression and relaxation, and the use of computers in diagnosis, as described in this paper, are just a few examples of the possible uses – offering advantages for patients and health professionals alike.

With regard again to prevention, I would like to suggest that there are four main ways in which the health care team can influence the development of adverse and maladaptive reactions and thus contribute significantly to preventive strategies and the promotion of sound mental health, by:
(i) anticipatory guidance; (ii) supportive intervention; (iii) early treatment; and (iv) referral – not necessarily to a psychiatrist. Many examples of alternative, beneficial sources of help appear in the chapters of this book.

(v) *Protocols for management*

Finally, I believe an important next step needed is for people involved in mental health to work together to devise *management protocols* for these distressing diseases and disorders. Protocols for asthma, hypertension and diabetes already use valid, objective procedures to measure peak expiratory flow, blood pressure and glycosylated haemoglobin. Why not use measures for anxiety and depression?

While it will not be so easy to develop protocols for psychiatric illness, I think we are in a position to make a start – and it is most important for our patients that we try. To be effective, teams must work to an agreed protocol: there must be guidelines for referral *back* to the GP, from specialist services. For example, endless counselling can prove counter-productive. Patients must not be allowed to fall between independent experts and get lost. Care must be continuous and consistent.

Conclusion

Mental ill-health is a major source of economic problems and human distress. The early recognition and appropriate management of emotional disorders – among which, anxiety and depression are two of the most common – require the application of special knowledge and skills; close co-operation between GPs and trained personnel from many backgrounds; and, most important, often long-term collaboration with the patients themselves. The judicious use of computer technology could help overcome problems with communication, often present in the early stages of professional consultation. Its role in the development and administration of management protocols, as is already possible with physical illness, also deserves further investigation. However, it must be remembered always that the computer complements, not replaces, doctor/patient contact and consultation.

References

1. Wright A F. A study of the presentation of somatic symptoms in general practice by patients with psychiatric disturbance. *British Journal of General Practice* 1990,**40**:459–463.
2. Goldberg D P. *Manual of the general health questionnaire.* Windor: NFER/Nelson, 1978.
3. Goldberg D P, Cooper B, Eastwood M R, Kedward H B, Shepherd M. A standardized psychiatric interview for use in community surveys. *Brit J Prev Soc Med* 1970;**24**:18–23.
4. Lewis G, Pelosi A J, Glover E, et al. The development of a computerised assessment for minor psychiatric disorder. *Psychol Med* 1988;**18**:737–745.
5. Eysenck H J, Eysenck SBG. *Manual of the Eysenck Personality Questionnaire.* London: Hodder and Stoughton, 1975.
6. Corney R H, Clare A W. The construction, development and testing of a self-report questionnaire to identify social problems. *Psychol Med* 1985;**15**:637–649.

Further reading

1. Wright A F. *Depression: a major problem in general practice.* In: Depression Information Folder (containing cassette tape for patients). London: Royal College of General Practitioners, 1990.
2. Poyser J. *Patient interviewing.* In: Sheldon M, Stoddart N, editors. Trends in general practice computing. London: Royal College of General Practitioners, 1985.

3. Carr A C, Ancill R J. Computers in psychiatry. *Acta Psychiatr Scand* 1983;**67**:137–143.

Address for contact

Dr Alastair Wright, 5 Alburne Crescent, Glenrothes KY7 5RE

7 Implications for General Practice Training and Education

PAUL FREELING, Professor of General Practice,
St George's Hospital Medical School, University of London

SUMMARY

Although both secondary and tertiary prevention of depression seem possible, prospects for primary prevention, despite encouraging developments (as described in this book) will become clearer with further elucidation of the natural history of affective disorders. Deficiencies identified in the care of depressive illness in general practice often originate in the failure to 'acknowledge' it to patients. 'Acknowledgement' is associated with the doctor's ability to show empathy, a quality best fostered by participation in case discussion in small groups – ie, in a method of learning and teaching basic to vocational training in general practice. Deficiencies in the care of anxiety often originate in failure to apply appropriate management. Methods of management can also be learnt during small-group-learning. A prevention approach, now being taught to medical students, can be fostered also in vocational training.

Background

My task is to discuss future approaches to medical education in general practice which might meet the requirements of a primary care service devoted to the aims of primary, secondary, and tertiary prevention of depression and anxiety. Undergraduate, vocational, and continuing education will be touched upon. A remit so vast is reassuring rather than daunting, because no-one can expect it to be met completely or be wholly supported by research-based evidence.

GPs are accustomed to tackling a job description too vast to be met. Indeed, we could be accused of writing our own job definition, and then using its comprehensiveness as an excuse to avoid assessment of how well we meet it! However, two components of the Job Definition of a GP[1] are particularly relevant for prevention-orientated practice:

(i) to 'integrate physical, psychological and social factors in considerations about health and illness';
(ii) to 'know how to intervene through treatment, prevention, and education to promote the health of patients and their families'.

The *New Contract*[2] also certainly pushes GPs towards taking a leading role in health promotion and preventive care. This and other changes make it necessary to determine what should be learnt about the discipline at various stages of the medical educational spectrum: ie, during undergraduate, continuing and vocational training.

Undergraduate education

Roughly half of the doctors in this country spend their working lives in general practice. At present, while general practice is likely to motivate students towards adopting a preventive approach, fewer find themselves able to put this into practice. How might this situation be improved?

Much teaching of undergraduates in general practice relies on case presentation in one-to-one and small-group settings. Students should be required to include a section on prevention in all case reports and to report the answers to three questions:

(i) Could this problem have been prevented?
(ii) Could intervention have been made earlier? If yes, where (and why) was the delay?
(iii) What steps could be taken to avoid recurrence of the problem or any delay?

The problems presented by patients to their GPs offer ample opportunity for these questions to be considered in the context of anxiety and depression and also in terms of primary, secondary and tertiary prevention (see Chapter 2). An understanding of these concepts and the model they offer, together with the rules which constrain the potential of screening techniques for primary and early secondary prevention, are an absolute requirement for all practising doctors, and essential learning for all medical students.

The model, its constraints, and their implications can be taught formally during basic science courses and demonstrated in most undergraduate clinical subjects. General practice is a particularly suitable arena, since its characteristics include not only adopting a preventive approach, but also, dealing with undifferentiated illness, using time as a management technique, and monitoring the development of people over their entire life span.

Medical students are exposed to a wide range of learning situations and teaching methods which can promote the principles of prevention; foster their perceptiveness; increase their social and interpersonal skills; and provide encouragement and support while they acquire self-knowledge and understanding. These efforts/opportunities are not limited to the departments of general practice and primary care: they extend throughout the curriculum. However, an interest in prevention, like an interest in social and inter-personal skills and in the development of self-knowledge, must pervade a school if it is to affect student (and staff) behaviour long term.

At St George's Hospital, more than 80 group practices each take our medical students for between 8 and 32 weeks a year. Some have done so for more than a decade. They work in close harmony with us in the central Department and accept a good deal of direction concerning their teaching objectives and methods.

Practices taking final-year students have the courage to allow them experience with patients which is supervised only at a distance. I feel privileged by our association and believe our students are very fortunate. Nevertheless, a group of some 320 GPs is likely to show heterogeneity similar to that of other like groups. The nature and extent of variability both of diagnosis and management within general practice has consequences for student learning, over and above the fundamental concern about its effect on patient care. Monitoring of the training process is thus essential.

In my seminars with clinical students, I am often initially concerned about the accuracy of the psychiatric diagnoses, the suitability of the management and follow-up described, and thus, the implications for effective prevention. However, I also read students' detailed case reports at the end of their first attachment to my department during their third to fourth year; I examine them orally at the end of their second attachment during their final year; and take part in their final exams. This contact reassures me about the extent of their knowledge base and the quality of their motivation. I am delighted by the perceptiveness of this intelligent seed-corn of our profession.

Continuing medical education

Variability in teaching skills is also likely to affect trainees in general practice. Other authors in this book believe that one cost-effective method of teaching GP trainees is to train the trainers in modes of behaviour related to basic psycho-therapeutic skills.

The economic logic of *teaching teachers* – in this context especially, of teaching them basic psycho-therapeutic skills (so akin to the basic skills needed in adult teaching) – and the benefits available from working in a skilfully-led group were adequately demonstrated during the Nuffield Courses organised by the Royal College of General Practitioners (RCGP) and from their evaluation[3]. The courses aimed to develop the knowledge, skills and attitudes of teachers who would teach trainers as well as those who would teach trainees. The philosophy of the courses was underpinned by several tenets, two of which are worth re-iterating:

(i) where patient care is concerned, that 'any increase in doctor-initiated, proactive, care brought the opportunity for planned whole-person care';
(ii) where principles of learning are concerned, that 'relevance, an identified need to know, is necessary for the learner and speeds learning'. Relevance is identified during clinical experience.

Psychiatry and learning in general practice

Undergraduate teaching should enable students to find out what medicine can do for patients; learning, inducing, and applying models which explain this; deducing what to do when faced with a problem, and acquiring basic knowledge, fundamental skills, and attitudes appropriate to future learning and patient care.

Continuing medical education consists more of learning how to do something fairly specific, the need for which has been identified from experience. A practitioner might need to be confronted with a particular experience or a trained teacher before he or she is able to identify needs rather than deny them.

Acknowledgement and management of depressive illness

Our studies[3,4,5] of GP variability in psychiatric matters have concentrated recently on depressive illness rather than anxiety. We have become more and more concerned about the acknowledgement and management by GPs of probable or definite Major Depressive Disorder as defined in the Research Diagnostic Criteria (RDC). This concern arises from three of our results:

(i) We have demonstrated *clearly* that treatment with tricyclic antidepressants is much more effective than placebo in patients for whom this diagnosis is correct. This does *not* mean that patients may be prescribed drugs and then ignored.

(ii) GPs fail to *acknowledge* half of the adults suffering from depression. We use the term *acknowledgement* because it seems that, although some GPs thought certain patients might be depressed, they did not make the minimum act of acknowledgement; ie, arrange to see them again within two weeks.

(iii) GPs have tended not to follow up and monitor acknowledged depressives.

The consultation process and depression: A research study

Our most recently completed study[4] compares the process of the consultations between a doctor and (i) an acknowledged depressive; (ii) an unacknowledged depressive; and (iii) a control patient matched for age and sex. Each doctor was asked to provide a video record of each type of consultation. The work, conducted by Dr André Tylee, whilst he was Mental Health Foundation Research Fellow in my Department, focused on the acknowledgement/non-acknowledgement of depression, deemed to be at least as severe as the RDC 'Probable Major' category. Tribute must be paid to the Foundation's adventurous decision to support training fellowships in psychiatry for GPs.

Some 50 GPs provided video tapes which were then analysed using the following schedules: Consultation Analysis, Triggers and Symptoms (CATS)[5]; and Consultation analysis, Behaviour and Styles (CABs). Each depressed patient when identified, had an extensive psychiatric research interview with Dr. Tylee and a follow-up session at three months with Heather Maughn, his research assistant. Comparisons of the research psychiatric interviews at diagnosis showed almost no differences between the illness of acknowledged and unacknowledged depressives; but comparisons of the three types of consultations showed remarkable differences in two parameters: (i) the presenting symptom; and (ii) the position of the first cue to a possible depressive illness in the sequence of symptoms mentioned.

Table 7.1 shows these items for the consultations with 19 control cases who were matched for age and sex to index unacknowledged cases, but who had a 30-item General Health Questionnaire (GHQ) score of less than five.

Seven controls mentioned one item from our fairly extensive list of 'depression cues'. Some of these could be explained as consequences of the presenting complaint or of the fact that the 30-item GHQ is not infallible. Patients do not always answer it honestly. However, only three of the cues appeared within the first five mentions – a sharp contrast to the acknowledged depressives (Table 7.2) for whom the first depression cue was also the presenting symptom

Table 7.1: Control cases

Presenting symptom	First verbal depression cue	Position of cue
1. Pain in thumb	none	–
2. Tetanus booster	none	–
3. Knee swelling	none	–
4. Coil change	none	–
5. Cough	none	–
6. Breast tenderness	none	–
7. Nasty taste	none	–
8. Sprained ankle	none	–
9. Lost voice	none	–
10. Lump in wound	none	–
11. Sheath burst	none	–
12. Numbness in hand	none	–
13. Vaginal burning	Wakes in night	17
14. Bit sick	Waking in night	2
15. Migraine	Gets on my nerves	9
16. Trouble with periods	Tired	4
17. Itching all over	Little sleep	6
18. Itch on leg	No energy	5
19. Dull arm ache	Feel so depressed	10

Table 7.2: Acknowledged depressives

Presenting symptom	First verbal depression cue	Position of cue
1. Depressed	–	1
2. So nervous	–	1
3. Redundancy worry	–	1
4. Cannot cope	–	1
5. Problem sleeping	–	1
6. Nerves gone	–	1
7. In a nervous state	–	1
8. No weight loss (diet)	–	1
9. Sore biopsy site	Tired	3
10. Funny thumb	Miserable	3
11. Leg pain	Can't be bothered	3
12. Breathing trouble	Frightened	3
13. Bad leg	Weight problem	3
14. Change of life	Depressed	4
15. Hip pain	Tension	5
16. Vomiting	Run down	7
17. Leg pulsation	Extremely tired	8
18. Abdominal pains	Worry	10
19. Bad sinusitis	Not happy	12
20. Abdominal pains	Boyfriend stress	20
21. Neck cyst	–	–
22. Weak leg	–	–

in 13 consultations; and only three offered the first cue later than 10 in the sequence of symptoms. The two correctly acknowledged cases who never gave a verbal cue should be noted: presumably examples of non-verbal communication!

Unacknowledged depressives (Table 7.3) showed a cluster of consultations – eight with no depression cue mentioned at all, and six mentioned quite late (>5). Most surprising perhaps were the seven consultations in which the first cue was mentioned very early, indeed in four, as the presenting symptom.

It is important to emphasise that the same doctors provided the consultation in each group of cases.

Even if these findings are not replicated in the full data set, there will still be a need to explain how a GP can fail to acknowledge depressive illness in, for instance, a woman in her early forties, whose opening statement is, 'I really am at point zero at the moment.' Who said later that she was, 'so depressed' and still later, 'so low'. Who, the next day, told a 'research doctor', about her recent divorce from a chronic alcoholic whose refusal to pay her maintenance meant she must work hard to pay her mortgage and support her 12-year-old, mentally-handicapped son and her 16-year-old boy, who had become 'a little difficult'. Who said openly that she was depressed.

Triggering behaviour: the importance of empathy

In four unacknowledged and 8 acknowledged consultations, the first depression cue was the opening (presenting) mention. For some reason, each patient felt able to volunteer the depressive cue immediately. Just as a trusting child

Table 7.3: *Unacknowledged depressives*

Presenting symptom	First verbal depression cue	Position of cue
1. Contractions	–	–
2. Fell off motor bike	–	–
3. Burning abdominal pain	–	–
4. Bronchial	–	–
5. Stomach pain	–	–
6. Foot rash	–	–
7. Catarrh	–	–
8. Knee pains	–	–
9. Pain passing urine	I feel low	24
10. Bellyaches	Miserable	14
11. Stomach cramps	Work worry	14
12. Bad throat	Feel down	10
13. Need antacid	Home stress	7
14. Skin rash	Lot of stress	5
15. At point zero	–	1
16. Not eating	–	1
17. Constipated	–	1
18. Extremely run down	–	1
19. Contraceptive request	Not any brighter	2
20. Hot flushes	Bad tempers	4
21. Bad throat	No energy	4

will run to outstretched arms, so these patients immediately volunteered intimate and distressing information about themselves. Since we could not identify triggering behaviour which might explain this action, we turned to our CABS schedule. This includes an empathy scale (Table 7.4) which we have modified from that described by Truax and Carkhuff[6]. It is a global rating of the degree to which the GP's responses have encouraged, or discouraged, the patient's attempts to communicate feeling during a consultation. The central rating 3, represents what seems to be a minimum acceptable performance – ie, professional, but not personal, warmth.

Table 7.5 shows our first results. For simplicity, the scale has been collapsed by combining empathy ratings 1 and 2 (tend to *discourage* patient communication), and 4 and 5 (tend to *encourage* patient communication).

These results, which include more than one consultation from some doctors, have been confirmed by re-analysis using our 39 'true' trios – ie, those in which the same doctors provided all the cases in each group. Even so, it is not possible to be certain of the direction of cause and effect – we are describing consultations, not doctors. It might be that the behaviours described are consequent upon a diagnosis having been formulated, rather than the behaviours resulting in information leading to the diagnosis. Doctors who were rated 'high' for empathy with some patients will have been rated low with others. There could be an element of choice in doctor behaviour: we found that several individual skills – eg, listening and use of silence – were often exhibited in consultations where depression was acknowledged. Obviously, the situation is more complicated than prediction from a single variable, even though some consistency has been introduced by selecting only patients experiencing probable major depressive illness.

Table 7.4: *Empathy scales*

Rating	GP's response to patient's expressed feelings
1	SUBTRACTS noticeably from expression of feeling
2	REDUCES expression of feelings
3	Professional but not personal warmth allows but DOES NOT ENCOURAGE expression of feelings
4	ADDS NOTICEABLY to patient's expression of feelings
5	ADDS SO SIGNIFICANTLY to expression of feelings that patient explores and reports self more deeply

Table 7.5 *Differences in empathy of doctors among acknowledged and unacknowledged depressed patients and emotionally normal controls*

Patient Group	Empathy Rating		
	1–2	3	4+5
	Per cent Doctors		
Controls	31	58	11
Acknowledged depressed	17	22	61
Unacknowledged depressed	49	33	18

Significance of difference among groups: P>0.0001

Our analyses are far from complete. Nevertheless, I am convinced that the quality of professional and personal warmth and the ability to encourage the expression of affect should be exhibited to *all* patients in *all* consultations in general practice. *The GP needs not only social and interpersonal skills, but, most important, self-knowledge:* objectives most likely to be achieved within an interactive, small group supervised by a skilled leader able to use a range of methods aimed at achieving specific tasks.

Developing empathy

The 'empathic' GP learns to be open to the emotions of others, unafraid of involvement, yet professionally responsible and able to tolerate his or her own uncertainty and helplessness. The clinical tasks best suited to developing these qualities and skills, are case discussion and a series of relatively long learning interviews with people needing help. I believe the models used to explain these interviews are much less important than the privilege of experiencing them: of sharing a room and a conversation with another human being who has come to you for help. Similarly, I believe the models underlying any case discussion are much less important than the extended intimacy with a patient and the consequent intimacy with a peer group which I consider to be absolute necessities.

The process again bears similarity to psychotherapy, for which time spent with the patient seems as good a predictor of benefit as the school of origin of the therapist. Close reading of reports on the learning of specified skills in small groups lends further credence to this belief. However, I spent five years in Balint training, and most of my teaching life since in small group teaching or teaching about small groups, so I would believe that, wouldn't I!

Managing anxiety

Discussion has focused so far on GPs and depressive illness. This is partly because, in depression, the faults in management seem to begin at identifying cues to the diagnosis: with anxiety, the faults seem further along the preventive process – namely, in selecting proper management. Where anxiety is concerned, the major immediate problem is to prevail on GPs to make the diagnosis at all, for they have been deprived of what must have seemed to be the miracle of the benzodiazepines.

I am extremely reluctant to prescribe anxiolytics because much of the anxiety presented to me seems to be associated with conflicts which need to be resolved, or with situations which will not disappear overnight. Consider for instance, anxiety associated with choosing between staying in a safe but boring job, or going back to full-time education as a mature university student. Using drugs to eliminate anxiety will remove at least part of the drive to resolve the conflict. Similarly, prescribing drugs for anxiety associated with having a violent husband, but providing no resources with which to leave him, seems more likely to produce dependency than sensible coping strategies. It is of no benefit to swap a situation full of conflict, but capable of resolution, for a life both stigmatised and damaged by taking benzodiazepines every day.

People differ in their responses to situations. In one sense, this reflects either their underlying personality or their learned behaviour. It seems essential that GPs should have readily-available alternatives to drug treatment which can seek to change learned behaviours.

Treatments: What, why, when and how?

In my clinical work, I find it useful to think of drug treatments as *WHAT* treatments, and alternative treatments as either *WHY* or *WHEN* and *HOW* treatments. My patients seem to understand their meaning without much difficulty.

WHY treatments aim at resolving conflict and represent forms of classical, non-directive counselling. This is a skill basic to general practice, and can be learned relatively easily in interactive small groups, particularly if further supervisory back-up is available. Its use is not limited to cases of anxiety. The implicit requirement for the person counselled to take responsibility for themselves will be highly conducive to tertiary prevention and thus to primary prevention of future episodes. New talking and listening techniques are constantly being developed.

'*WHEN* do you have your anxiety symptoms?' is usually a more helpful approach to use with anxious patients. Doctor and patient can then explore just what those symptoms stop the patient from doing, or whether more positive avoidance behaviour is provoked. People can find it difficult to leave their homes, enter crowded shops, or use public transport: some have to check constantly in an attempt to dispel anxiety. Once such specific situations have been identified, patients can learn to overcome their fears.

HOW therapies are my name for desensitisation techniques. They are aimed at the disabling phobic fears which patients may present to GPs, at first as unfocused anxieties. Many patients can be helped so simply that referral is unnecessary, but familiarity with the principles of desensitisation and the range of techniques is essential for all practising GPs. The experience may even help GPs with their own anxieties which would otherwise hinder intimate communications with their patients.

Vocational training and the pre-registration year

There are several reasons for only sketching in the possible effects on vocational training of requiring all GPs to take a preventive approach to anxiety and depression. A major reason is that the duty of teaching trainees the importance of a preventive approach to these conditions is laid on us already. The implication, therefore, is simply a matter of 'getting on with it'. Obviously, there are other important things to say.

The *purpose* of vocational education is to build on the foundations provided by the undergraduate curriculum. Trainees should be taught *when* to do *what*. If opportunity affords, they should be taught *how* to do *some* of it. Anxiety and depression are sufficiently important to receive a fair portion of the time allocated to vocational training. But what is a fair portion of a single trainee year?

Trainees must leave their vocational period aware that there is a lot more yet to be learnt. Their future partners should realise that they are receiving a doctor prepared for development – *not* one fully mature.

New principals interested in learning new skills should be encouraged to work in small groups led by an experienced trainer. I believe that the best way to develop and maintain empathy is to use forms of case discussion in professionally-led, small groups. It is certainly the only way to learn to understand patients. The material for case discussion should vary – from case reports to the use of audio- and video-feedback. This will improve specific skills. Finally, GPs should not be ashamed of using old-fashioned rote-memorising to learn the component symptoms which make up syndromes with proven modes of management.

Whether we are considering anxiety and depression, or asthma, otitis media, diabetes or osteo-arthritis, there seems to me to be a risk that GP trainers and course organisers might be fighting yesterday's battles and not seeking to build on changes already in place in the undergraduate curriculum. Because the curriculum varies from school to school, GP trainers need to assess the skills, strengths and weaknesses of their trainees, and respond accordingly. As a corollary, I know that all my fellow heads of Departments of General Practice would welcome adequate feedback. I am fortunate to work in the only medical school in the Region; GPs who teach my students are often later their trainers and we all get good feed-back.

Conclusion

I cannot resist a little acrobatic riding on my twin hobby horses in any discussion of education in general practice. First, why have we not gone flat out for five years vocational training giving three years dedicated learning to a job which requires a high level of skill and personal growth? Second, why do we perpetuate an archaic administrative division between Departments of General Practice on one hand and Postgraduate Advisers on the other?

Perhaps the two are causally linked? Perhaps we perpetuate these anomalies so that, when faced by challenges of the nature posed by chapters in this book, we GPs can respond with our species-specific cry: 'If only we had more time!'.

References

1. Freeling P. *A workbook for trainees in general practice.* London: Wright, 1983.

2. Department of Health. *General practice in the National Health Service: the 1990 contract: the Government's programme for changes to GP's terms of service and renumeration system.* London: Department of Health, 1989.

3. Freeling P, Barry S. *In-service training: a study of the Nuffield courses of the Royal College of General Practitioners.* Windsor: NFER-Nelson, 1982.

4. Tylee A, Freeling P. The recognition, diagnosis and acknowledgement of depressive disorders by general practitioners. In: *'Depression: An Integrated Approach'* London: Mental Health Foundation, 1989:216–231

5. Tylee A, Freeling P. Consultation analysis by triggers and symptoms (CATS). A new objective technique for studying consultations. *Family Practice*, 1987:4(4):260–265.

6. Truax C B, and Carkhuff R R. *Towards effective counselling and psychotherapy.* Chicago: Aldine, 1967.

Further reading

1. Leeuwenhorst Working Party. The general practitioner in Europe. *J R Coll Gen Pract* 1977:27:117

2. Bloom B S. *Taxonomy of educational objectives. Handbook 1: cognitive domain.* London: Longman 1956.

3. Bloom B S, Krathwohl D S and Masia B B. *Taxonomy of educational objectives. Handbook 2: affective domain.* London: Longman, 1964.

4. Royal College of General Practitioners. *The future general practitioner – learning and teaching.* British Medical Journal 1972: 225–6.

Address for contact

Professor Paul Freeling, Department of General Practice, St George's Hospital Medical School, Blackshaw Road, London SW17

8 Crisis Support: Utilising Resources

JENNIFER NEWTON, Prevention Research Officer, MIND, London

SUMMARY

Three criteria can be used to define 'good practice' in prevention: current understanding of aetiology must be used to define a high-risk group, and to plan a strategy likely to reduce that risk; the support offered should help people find their own solutions; and the intervention should draw on and strengthen support available from relatives, friends, voluntary groups and other 'front-line' carers. The implications of these criteria are traced, using a psychosocial model of depression. Lack of care in childhood is one of the antecedent factors linked to a raised risk of depression in adulthood. Families with marked parenting problems, or adolescents leaving care could therefore be targeted. Voluntary befriending initiatives are one particularly important innovation. In general practice, risk of depression is most readily identifiable at the point where an individual is failing to cope with a psychosocial crisis. He or she needs information, advice, counselling, and/or practical support. Ways in which practices could enhance their support in these terms are discussed.

Background

The prevention of mental illness was the subject of my research for a number of years. In 1983, MIND commissioned me to prepare

(i) a review of research and theory relevant to the prevention of depression and schizophrenia[1]; and
(ii) a review and description of examples of good preventive practice[2].

This work left me with three over-riding conclusions about the characteristics of effective prevention-oriented health services and of those features which constitute 'good practice' in the delivery of preventive care. To be effective, such services must:

(i) Target the people known to be most at risk of a particular disorder. The reasons for their increased risk should be well understood and preventive intervention programmes influenced by that knowledge (ie, from a credible aetiological model).
(ii) Help people take control of their own lives, without inadvertently increasing their dependence on other people's support or expertise.

(iii) Make the maximum use of voluntary, community and 'natural' caring networks (ie, family and friends), and should not threaten resources for secondary care.

The following discussion summarises why I believe these criteria are important, and provides examples of, and suggestions for, good preventive practice based on them.

Targeting high-risk groups

The disease model

My first premise is that intervention is based on a credible 'disease' model and targeted at people known to be at high risk of the disorder in question. This model is appropriate for the prevention and management of mental, as well as physical, illness and may be complemented by a health promotion model. Figure 8.1 illustrates a simplistic disease model.

Intervention may be directed at A, B, C, or D, but prevention will be most effective if the antecedent factors A and B are known and can be addressed. When knowledge of A, B and C is limited, intervention can focus only on D, and treatment arranged as soon as the disorder is identified. When something is known about bodily mechanisms and behaviour which precede the onset of a disorder, intervention can be planned earlier (at C): as when routine screening (eg, for cervical cancer or raised blood pressure levels) reveals an abnormality (pre-cancerous cells or hypertension, respectively).

The effectiveness of such screening programmes can be improved if more information about antecedent factors is available. However, there may be ethical and practical issues to consider. For example, because several risk factors associated with cervical cancer are well known, women who have a history of wart virus or who smoke could be screened more often than is recommended for those considered to be less at risk. Likewise, men over 40 and people with a family history of heart disease could have their blood pressure checked more frequently. Innovations such as introduction of the recently-proposed patient-held, personal health record and health summary card[3] might facilitate the wider use of such strategies.

Figure 8.1 *Disease model and possibilities for prevention*

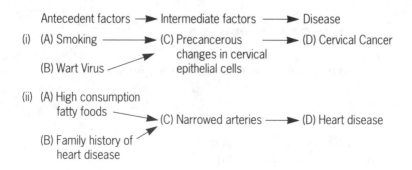

For some common physical disorders, it is possible to address factors A and B through health promotion strategies directed at the general population: eg, against smoking, a high consumption of saturated fats, alcohol misuse and lack of exercise; the management of stress, etc. England's national *'Look after your Heart!'* healthy lifestyle's programme[4], introduced in 1987 to combat the country's chief cause of premature death and morbidity – coronary heart disease – is such a strategy.

Health promotion strategies

A health promotion strategy which effectively focuses on any factor known to have a causal role in a disorder and which encourages the *whole* population to change their habits becomes rational for four reasons:

First — The target factor has been identified by research as having a causal role in a specific disorder.

Second — The disorder(s) to which these factors contribute affect either (i) many people (eg, coronary heart disease); or (ii) fewer numbers, but with usually fatal results; and/or the potential for spread is significant (eg, AIDS).

Third — These factors are *important enough* to warrant attention and the necessary strategies are *straightforward enough* and *cheap enough* to mount on a population-wide scale.

Fourth — No-one – including people *not* at risk of developing a specific disorder – will be harmed by the measures.

If any of these criteria do not apply, it may be considered wiser and cheaper to wait for people to show early symptoms of trouble and then treat them. For mental illness, the strategies required are usually neither straightforward enough nor cheap enough to make a general population health promotion approach a realistic option (although more child care provision, job sharing and lower unemployment could be justified in these terms. And of course there are some general strategies that we now take for granted which have a good preventive effect on mental as well as physical health, such as good antenatal care, and sex education for teenagers to prevent unwanted pregnancies). But in terms of approaches specific to mental illness, I would argue that it is *usually* better to use the best disease model available to identify another causal factor; to thus narrow the risk group; and to then provide the measure(s) or message(s) appropriate for that smaller group.

Causal factors in depression

The aetiological model for depression which I have found most useful is one evolved from well-respected research done by George Brown, Tirril Harris and their colleagues[5,6] (see Chapter 3). This describes three main sets of aetiological factors:

(i) *provoking agents*,
(ii) *vulnerability factors*, and
(iii) *symptom-formation factors*.

Only (i) and (ii) are relevant to prevention: symptom-formation factors affect the *form* the depression takes, rather than whether or not it occurs.

Provoking agents are major psychosocial *difficulties* present for at least two years (eg, caring for a relative suffering from a distressing chronic condition such as advanced dementia; or living in markedly substandard accommodation) and severe, threatening *events* (eg, a disabling accident to, or suicide of, a close relative). Both can occur together, and an event which follows a long period of difficulty can be particularly traumatic.

Most depression is preceded by such stresses, but most people who experience them do *not* get depressed to an extent comparable with the severity seen by psychiatrists working in outpatient clinics. Although they will feel quite depressed, they will cope with support from partners, relatives and/or friends (see Chapter 3). Some people thus appear to be more vulnerable than others to clinical depression.

Vulnerability factors are closely linked to the quality of past and current support experienced by an individual. In a crisis, the presence of one person with whom the individual has a close, confiding relationship – often a marital partner or special friend – and who can provide practical and emotional support, is most important. Throughout childhood, the quality of support received from parents or parent substitutes is also crucial. A low level of control, combined with indifference – even abuse – and experienced for at least a year, can increase vulnerability to depression. George Brown and his colleagues[7] have shown that such lack of care in childhood is linked to an increased vulnerability to depression in adulthood through two possible pathways:

(a) directly, by affecting personality characteristics such as *helplessness*; and
(b) more indirectly, by the effects of experiences which can follow poor parenting: substitute care arrangements, institutional care, unintended early pregnancy, continued low social class status, stressful adult lifestyle, and poor personal support.

Possibilities for preventive action

This model of depression offers several possibilities for preventive action. Two important options available are to:

(i) *target people* who are experiencing a distressing event or long-term difficulty when they present in general practice. Those who seem not to have the resources to cope can be offered more help (Stage C: Figure 8.1). Often, those vulnerable to depression will already have a number of symptoms, as depression typically follows a provoking agent within a matter of weeks. Early diagnosis and appropriate intervention (ie, at stage D) then offer the best results. David Goldberg (see Chapter 4) and Linda Gask (Chapter 5) describe how skilled interview techniques can help practitioners detect emotional disorders in primary care settings at the earliest stage possible. Professor Freeling (see Chapter 7) emphasises the importance of empathy exhibited by the interviewer.

or

(ii) *intervene earlier*, providing support for people likely to be vulnerable to depression. An examination of the links between lack of care in childhood and adult depression reveals some of the possibilities for intervention.

Early intervention: targeting children at risk

By taking just one major antecedent (vulnerability) factor – *lack of care in childhood* – it is possible to see what three of these options might be.

(i) *Support for mothers and babies*
Parent-child difficulties can sometimes be predicted – even during the short time spent in hospital following childbirth. A formalised screening programme can ensure that all women about whom the midwives feel concerned are discussed at weekly meeting of professionals in child health. Some might be thought to need special help, but at the very least, such a service can ensure that the appropriate GP and health visitor are alerted to the midwife's concerns. They can then plan to visit the family more frequently. Ounsted and colleagues[8] reported that this simple strategy produced a decline in the number of cases of serious child abuse.

(ii) *The parent-child relationship*
Families where marked parenting problems exist can be offered a planned programme of support. Continuing difficulties in the relationship between parent and child mean that both parties are lacking an important source of self-esteem. Improvements in the relationship will reduce the vulnerability of the child in the long-term and should also alleviate symptoms of depression or anxiety often present in the parent.

In the United Kingdom, projects run by voluntary agencies – eg, NEWPIN and HOME-START (see Chapter 13A) – befriend women with young children in their own homes. Keith Beswick and Pauline Richardson (see Chapter 10A) describe how a support group and drop-in centre can help mothers, with similar responsibilities and problems, to share their problems, and gain new ways of coping with their difficulties.

(iii) *Young people leaving 'care'*
If serious parenting problems are not prevented or significantly relieved, children may be placed in the care of local authorities. A prime opportunity to reduce the obvious vulnerability of this group occurs as they leave institutions or foster care to set up homes of their own. The poor quality support recieved throughout much of their childhood, and the possible lack of close, caring relationships or sound practical support in their current living circumstances leave them very little to fall back on as they attempt to establish satisfying lives as independent adults.

Statistics indeed reflect the difficulties they experience. Articles in 'Roof'[9], (the magazine of the housing charity, Shelter), have reported a disturbingly high rate of homelessness among them. David Quinton and Michael Rutter[10] have illustrated the very high rates of premarital pregnancy among girls leaving care, and the increased likelihood of them then experiencing difficulties parenting their own children. These findings have profound implications for ways in which local authorities and Social Services should be supporting young people in their care.

Maximising personal autonomy

Research in the United States, on pre-school education for disadvantaged children[11], has shown that the more a mother is able to improve her child's behaviour or educational skills (and to see *herself* as responsible for these improvements), the longer the improvements tend to last. The improvements are mutually reinforcing: as a child's behaviour improves, the mother sees herself in control again. In turn, the increased care and attention motivates the child to please her, and this increased responsiveness gives the mother more pleasure (and vice versa). In other words, the *mother must be helped to help herself*.

Helping people to take control over their own lives will affect both the content of the intervention and *the way* in which that support is delivered. Traditional client-helper relationships might need to be avoided, and for this reason, befriending mechanisms have much to offer. Improvements associated with professional support may be attributed more to the skills of the expert than to those of the mother herself.

Support and experiences which enable individuals to feel that they have the power to influence their own circumstances for the better, provide crucial protection against depression, and this has been recognised for decades by influential research workers[12–15]. For these reasons, I believe that good preventive practice should include measures which help people take control of their lives.

Choosing and using resources

General principles

Influencing the support available to, and the style of thinking of individuals might be neither cheap nor straightforward. If it is not, intervention must be *targeted*. If the targeting can be precise – eg, for people who (i) although currently well, do suffer from severe, recurrent attacks of depression, or (ii) already have clear symptoms present – expensive professional time, as is used for counselling, can be justified. If successful, the initial high cost should be balanced by the reduced need for long-term care and/or, use of secondary care services.

Intervention on a broader scale (ie, where targeting is inaccurate or impossible) must make use of less expensive resources. Many of the preventive hopes cherished by the Community Mental Health Centres (CMHC) Movement in the United States foundered when it became apparent that trying to cater for all areas of human need with professional resources was like trying to drink the ocean[16]! There can *never* be sufficient professional resources to meet all needs. Preventive work thus demands the innovative use of para-professionals, of community groups, of natural caring networks, and collaboration between existing services.

The innovative use of resources, support which helps people take control over their own lives, and targeting are the three crucial components of good preventive practice.

Supporting people through crises: GP options

When people who are (or who are not) coping with a recent traumatic event, or long-term difficulties come to the surgery, what can the GP do?

Other contributors here have suggested how the detection and management of depression can be improved during the 10-minute interview (see Chapters 4, 5 and 7). However, GPs can use resources other than their own expertise. People with psychosocial problems usually want information; a chance to talk things through; and practical assistance.

(i) *Keeping informed/providing information*
A wealth of printed material and other aids is produced by reliable sources such as the Health Education Authority, and numerous non-statutory organisations which work on behalf of people with specific health or social needs (eg, MIND: the National Association for Mental Health; CRUSE: the bereavement support agency; NACAB: the National Association of Citizens Advice Bureaux; and the Alzheimer's Disease Society). Perhaps more of these could be made available to patients, or at least, patients could be informed of their publications and services (eg, help lines). Clare Pace, for example, describes how to set up a health library in the practice waiting area (Chapter 12A); Robert Gann (Chapter 12B) indicates how a readily-accessible, local data base, such as the *Help for Health* project in Southampton, can benefit both health professionals and their clients.

Many practices could improve their use of surgery waiting rooms for health promotion. Why not, for instance, complement 'popular' magazines with health-oriented journals; show short video films on health topics; and loan out health videos, and audio cassettes – as also advocated by Clare Pace? The local library could be invited to arrange displays of suitable publications in the health centre's main waiting area, changing them every few weeks – just as is already done in many homes for the elderly.

(ii) *'Talking through' problems*
People who are emotionally distressed often need the opportunity to talk through major social problems or relationship difficulties, and if necessary, to receive counselling.

GPs have a range of resources to call upon if they have exhausted their own time or expertise. They may, for example, organise a counselling service within the practice itself (see Chapter 9C and 9D); establish links with counsellors in local voluntary agencies (see Chapter 9B); arrange for a psychologist, social worker or community psychiatric nurse to be attached to the practice (see Chapter 9A); or work with other professional services, such as crisis support or community mental health teams (see Chapters 11A and B).

(iii) *Mobilising practical support*
GPs can mobilise practical support for patients whose needs have been clearly defined. Local community and voluntary organisations are the key resources

here, but practitioners need to determine not only the presence of such groups, but also, the type and quality of support they can deliver.

Patients' needs vary widely. A nearly-blind mother, who is becoming very depressed because she is unable to transport her children to social activities and is feeling their resentment, is likely to benefit from contact with a Good Neighbours scheme. Parents whose baby is found to be mentally handicapped could receive support from the local MENCAP group. A socially-isolated mother with young children might welcome the friendship and practical help offered by a HOME-START volunteer. A person, becoming or already dependent on tranquillisers, may find hope and help with breaking the addiction, through contact with a group which specialises in such problems (see Chapter 13B).

These 'prescriptions' can play a crucial role in the prevention of emotional disorders; in limiting their often widespread adverse affects; or at least, in preventing acute distress from developing into a chronic depressive condition.

Caryle Steen, in her description of general practice in North West London (see Chapter 14), outlines how a practice team can form effective, personalised, working relationships with neighbourhood support agencies. Key figures from local groups and organisations are invited to meet the practice staff at a team meeting; to explain the nature and functions of their work; and to discuss possible referral mechanisms. In this way, the team gains an accurate idea of the range and quality of support available in the area. A practice wishing to set up similar close links with their community could perhaps make the practice manager responsible for finding out what organisations and other resources are available locally, and for arranging meetings with them. Two-way benefits may arise from these links if the practice is also able to offer support to the group(s).

Conclusion

GPs and their colleagues in primary care practice can improve the preventive mental health care of their patients in many ways – without exceeding existing financial constraints. These measures mostly entail innovative use of the many local and national resources available which can provide information, advice, counselling or practical support to people coping with distressing circumstances. GPs might also consider becoming involved in collaborative strategies to support young families where marked problems in the parent-child relationship are suspected. Such action could reduce the children's vulnerability to depression in adult life.

References

1. Newton J. *Preventing mental illness*. London: Routledge, 1988.
2. Newton J. *Preventing mental illness in practice*. London: Routledge, 1992.
3. Richards T. Patient-held records. *BMJ* 1991;**302**:611.
4. Look after your heart. *Health Trends* 1987;**19**(2):special issue.

5. Brown G W, Harris T O. *Social origins of depression*. London: Routledge, 1978.

6. Brown G W. *Depression: a radical social perspective*. In: Herbert K R, Paykel E S, editors. Depression: an integrated approach. Oxford: Heinemann Medical Books, 1989.

7. Brown G W, Harris T O, Bifulco A. *Long-term effect of early loss of parent*. In: Rutter M, Izard C, Read P, editors. Depression in young people: developmental and clinical perspectives. New York: Guildford Press, 1985.

8. Ounsted C, Roberts J C, Gordon M, Milligan B. Fourth goal of perinatal medicine. *BMJ* 1982;**284**:879–882.

9. Grosskurth A. From care to nowhere. *Roof* 1984;July/August:11–14.

10. Rutter M L, Quinton D, Liddle C. *Parenting in two generations: looking backwards and looking forwards*. In: Madge N, editor. Families at risk. London: Heinemann Educational, 1983.

11. Bronfenbrenner U. *Is early intervention effective?* In: Guttentag M, Struening E L, editors. Handbook of evaluation research. Beverly Hills: Sage, 1975.

12. Bowlby J. *Attachment and loss: Vol 3: Loss*. London: Hogarth Press, 1980.

13. Beck A T. *The diagnosis and management of depression*. Philadelphia: University of Pennsylvania Press, 1973.

14. Seligman M E P. *Helplessness*. San Francisco: Freeman, 1975.

15 Quinton D, Rutter M. *Parenting behaviour of mothers raised 'in care'*. In: Nicol A R, editor. Practical lessons from longitudinal studies. Chichester: Wiley, 1983.

16. Leighton A. *Caring for mentally ill people: psychological and social barriers in a historical context*. Cambridge: Cambridge University Press, 1982.

Address for contact

Dr Jennifer Newton, Health Education Authority, Hamilton House, Mabledon Place, London WC1H 9TX.

9 Counselling in General Practice

A Options for Action: Clinical Psychology

MEREDITH ROBSON, Clinical Psychologist,
Charing Cross Hospital, London

SUMMARY

This article describes the work of a clinical psychologist in a general practice setting. It introduces the main features of the cognitive behavioural approach to therapy which make it suitable for the psychologist, general practitioner, or other primary health care staff to use in the brief time available for standard patient consultations. It is particularly suitable for disorders which are primarily anxiety based. Clinical assessment aided by information from patient diaries leads to individual treatment plans which incorporate specific skills and techniques which can be learnt and used by the patient. Patient and therapist can monitor progress and homework can be assisted by reference books, tapes and instruction manuals. The case history of a man suffering from bouts of anxiety and depression is presented to illustrate how the techniques may be used effectively.

Background

My ideas about how a clinical psychologist might work with a general practice team are based on personal experience and research findings gained from three positions:

(i) Three years research at Yateley Medical Centre, Surrey with Dr Richard France which investigated the therapeutic efficacy and cost-effectiveness of clinical psychology in primary care[1]. A total of 429 patients, originally thought by the GP to have psychological problems, were randomly assigned to either the GP or the psychologist. Fifty per cent of the patients referred suffered from anxiety and ten per cent of those from depression. (The remainder had other psychological problems such as interpersonal or occupational difficulties or habit disorders). The results showed significant differences during the first six months of treatment. Patients seeing the psychologist improved more rapidy ($p = 0.02$ over 6 months). They used significantly less psychotropic medication ($p = 0.01$ over 12 months) and paid fewer visits to the GP ($p = 0.0008$ to 6 months).

(ii) Two years as a therapist at the University of London Health Centre where many staff and students are referred for help with anxiety related to study and examinations.

(iii) Current research at Charing Cross Hospital, London, which is designed to test whether patients normally seen by their GP will travel to a nearby hospital for a service identical to that provided by the home practice: ie, they will be seen within one week for short periods, and have a choice of appointment times – before or after work. Results show that they are willing to attend the hospital and, as a result, a service can be offered to five local practices. The programme is separate from the usual hospital service and side-steps the waiting list.

Cognitive behavioural therapy

Cognitive behavioural therapy offers several advantages over traditional psychoanalytic therapy in general practice. The sessions are generally brief and of short-term duration. The aim is to modify the patient's thoughts and behaviour without necessarily understanding the often deep-seated psychological reasons for it. The main features of this approach are:

(i) *Assessment*. The patient sometimes has a specific medical condition but more often, is referred with vague, ill-defined symptoms or feelings of anxiety. The assessment procedure tries to describe their nature, frequency and intensity – ie, make a *functional analysis* of the problem. The likely development, current maintaining factors and consequences of the problem are looked for. This process may take one or several sessions and information is obtained from the use of individually-designed diaries, questionnaires or behavioural tests completed between sessions. Therapists quite often go out with patients to observe what happens; or, if patients are obsessional, they may make them undertake certain activities and examine the results.

(ii) *Individual treatment plans*. An individually-tailored treatment plan is developed from the information gathered and negotiated by the patient and the therapist together. The programme is flexible and subject to modification according to further information received. Other members of the primary health care team, friends and relatives often assist with therapy. For example, in the treatment of agoraphobia (fear of open spaces) relatives or friends may assist patients in a graded programme of exposure to situations which are being avoided because they elicit fear and anxiety. The psychologist might simply be required to help decide weekly goals and then examine the monitoring sheets and personal diaries prepared by the patient, and his or her supporters, as treatment continues and progress is made.

(iii) *Treatment skills and techniques*. Treatment techniques and skills which have been experimentally evaluated or which can be developed for a particular patient and then tested empirically are taught. For example, the control of hyperventilation is a technique often needed by patients suffering from anxiety. Others include interviewing skills, relaxation, challenging of negative thoughts and depression, and the prevention of unwanted responses to obsessional behaviour. The skills are important in terms of prevention as well as modification of current problems as they are transferable and may be used in various situations. They may be called upon at a later date to deal with similar or related problems. For example, relaxation techniques can be used when going to the dentist or travelling on public transport – not surprisingly perhaps, often on the London Underground. Cognitive techniques may be used to avert recurrent depression.

(iv) *Monitoring and evaluating therapy.* Therapy is closely monitored and can be effectively evaluated. Both these features allow therapists and patients to gain a better understanding of the nature of the illness and how best it might be managed. More realistic management/treatment programmes can be tested in this way with both therapist and patient gaining confidence from subsequent progress.

(v) *Books, tapes and instruction manuals.* These are often included in treatment programmes. Although useful on their own[2] they are most effective when used to supplement the work done in clinical sessions, the patient being able to use them for reference between appointments and after treatment has ended.

(vi) *Short interventions.* Interventions are often frequent and brief (eg, 15–30 minutes per week over a one-month period). Assessment may be spread over several brief appointments. Subsequent sessions may also be brief – one lasting only 10 minutes being needed to check a patient's progress and decide the next goal. Complex probems require more and longer sessions, each lasting approximately 60 minutes, but spread over six months. There are no fixed rules; the programmes are determined by the nature of the illness and the patient's response.

The research at Yateley[1], where the duration of treatment was recorded for 200 patients over a two-year period, showed that the average total time spent with a patient was two hours and thirty-four minutes. This time involved approximately four clinical visits. Similar findings have been replicated by colleagues at a local health centre near Charing Cross, where only three sessions was the average (S Thornton, personal communication).

The flexibility in the duration and nature of clinical contact may be best described by example: a child with a bed-wetting problem might need only five minutes of the therapist's time to bring in his diary, have it checked, and receive a pat on the back. Some problems require more therapeutic time than is feasible in the GP surgery. However, the patient will then be referred to the hospital-based psychology department or, if appropriate, to voluntary organisations or self-help groups. In both instances the psychologist's role is facilitatory.

(vii) *Collaboration* with GPs, other health professionals, and voluntary agencies ensures that patients receive specific and often, ongoing support. The help given ranges from the prescription of medication to complementary psychological assessment. This sharing and working together promotes better understanding and the development of professional support networks which benefit both patients and members of the primary care team.

Case history

The following case history illustrates some of the points made above.

At the *first session* a 37-year-old man, referred by his GP, complained of bouts of anxiety and depression, lasting several days to several weeks, which had occurred over the past two years. He had tried anti-depressant medication for several months without benefit so had decided to stop it. The depression, which had begun after he changed his job had increased in frequency during the previous six months. When depressed, the man's fears centred on what would happen if he lost his job or was too ill to work. These thoughts became 'catastrophic'. He became lethargic and pessimistic. He believed he would lose personal status, his house, his girlfriend, and his job. He doubted that he would find alternative work.

He felt worse at home when not doing anything, and at the end of the session, he suggested that his depression was most probably triggered by pressure of work and maintained by the negative thoughts. He also made frequent statements which provoked anxiety symptoms and feelings of guilt: eg, 'I *must* succeed!', 'I *must* get this finished at all costs!'; 'If things go wrong others blame me and I am a reject.' He was asked to keep a record, for a week, of these thoughts and feelings and of the situations in which they occurred.

At the *second session* (3 weeks later), as a result of his notes, our hypothesis was modified. The records showed that pressure both at work or at home, and periods of leisure time with nothing to do, all provoked anxiety and hyperventilation. This aggravated the negative thought cycle and depression. The man learned to control his breathing and to fill his free time more constructively. He was very worried at that stage that if he relaxed more and cared less he would eventually not care about anything at all! Would never get up in the morning! Again he was shown how he could accept the blame for things, relax a little, and look at the consequences.

By the *third session* (3 weeks later) he reported considerable improvement. This he attributed to his ability to control his breathing and thus the unpleasant symptoms and consequences of hyperventilation. However, his diary showed that he had never been able to enjoy free time because he felt he ought to be doing something. He felt bad whether he worked or not.

The *fourth and final session* (2 months later) concentrated on longterm planning; on setting aside amounts of intentional free time where he could begin to challenge his previously-held beliefs and free himself of further anxiety and guilt.

Outcome

He asked for a follow-up appointment two months after the third session to assess his progress. This was arranged and indeed, he had at the time of writing, continued to improve. His problem assessment scales show a significantly reduced score.

Conclusion

A trained clinical psychologist, working in general practice and in close collaboration with colleagues from the primary care team, can, by using well-founded and tried techniques – in this case cognitive behavioural therapy – contribute significantly to the management of emotional disorders, particularly anxiety.

References

1. Robson M H, France R, Bland M. Clinical psychologist in primary care: controlled clinical and economic evaluation. *Br Med J* 1984;**288**,1805–8.

2. Marks I M. *Living with fear: understanding and coping with anxiety*. London: McGraw Hill 1978.

Further reading

France R, Robson M. *Behaviour therapy in primary care: a practical guide*. London: Chapman and Hall, 1986.

Address for contact

Meredith Robson, Department of Psychology, Charing Cross Hospital, Fulham Palace Road, London W6.

9 Counselling in General Practice

B Options for Action: A Social Worker's Point of View

MARY BURKE, The Surgery,
241 Westbourne Grove, LONDON W11 2SE.

SUMMARY

The process of introducing a social worker/counsellor successfully as a member of the primary care team is described. The overall result was that a new approach to the management of patients was introduced, the quality of patient care improved, and team members felt a greater sense of satisfaction in their work. The social worker/counsellor works effectively with a wide variety of health-related social problems and brings particular expertise in counselling skills, knowledge of and liaison with local resources, and networking skills. There is enormous scope for developing social work/counselling support services for vulnerable and needy patients in collaboration with colleagues in the primary health care team, and in the local community and professional network.

Background

A social worker attached to general practice

In 1981, the Kensington Westminster branch of the Family Welfare Association, an independent social work agency, assisted by the local MIND Centre, set up a pilot scheme which attached a social worker (myself) for a period of six months, to a local group general practice. This practice, which cares for 8,000 patients, has a catchment area which covers the inner-city, multi-racial areas of North Kensington and Bayswater. Both districts have large numbers of single people of all ages, living in bedsitting rooms; homeless families living in temporary accommodation – in bed-and-breakfast hostels; and many people with problems of drug addiction and alcoholism. The surgery estimates that over 70 per cent of its patients consult their GP for emotional, social and psychiatric reasons, rather than physical illness. At the time of my appointment, the attached social worker saw patients referred from the practice at the social work agency situated about five minutes walk from the surgery.

Monitoring progress

For the duration of the pilot scheme, meetings, chaired by the MIND representative, and attended by the GPs and myself were held each six weeks to discuss problems as they arose. These meetings contributed greatly to the final success of the scheme.

Patient management

A group, which at first involved only three GPs and a social worker, met for one and a half hours each week at the surgery to discuss patient-referrals, the results of social-work assessment, and specific points of management affecting selected patients. This group was extended to include a psychologist, a community psychiatric nurse (CPN), trainee GPs and social workers, and, occasionally, a health visitor or representative from a local agency (eg psychiatric day centre).

The patient review group provided valuable experience in multi-disciplinary work for its members, as well as a practical resource which helped improve the quality of patient care. For example, when patients and their background history were discussed, members learnt much about each other's professional roles, skills and ways of working. The advantage of this insight was evident when GPs' prescribing habits were debated. Other members of the group considered that the use of medication was often excessive. The GPs admitted that they wrote more prescriptions when they 'did not know what else to do'. Prescriptions thus often met the doctors' rather than the patients' needs.

A small, but significant, decrease in the number of prescriptions issued occurred gradually when the doctors were offered an acceptable option – a psycho-therapeutically trained counsellor to whom they could refer patients. Someone whom they had learnt to trust; someone easily accessible to them. The group experience also made the doctors better able to tolerate uncertainty. They became more confident and proud of their professional development. The newly-acquired interviewing and listening skills enabled them to explore a patient's presenting problems more sensitively and effectively. In this way, a whole new approach to the management of patients was introduced. In turn, other members of the group learned how GPs were often exposed to very high levels of stress in their daily work. This acknowledgement by their colleagues provided the GPs with much needed support.

Health-related social problems for the counsellor

A great variety of health-related social problems prompted referrals to the counsellor. They often involved a mixture of unsatisfactory family relationships and social circumstances and emotional difficulties. The following case history provides a typical example.

Mr A

Mr A, a 47-year old Asian, was referred by his GP, suffering from severe stress and anxiety. He, his wife and their two daughters, aged five and three years, lived in overcrowded accommodation. His wife was having a difficult third pregnancy, and his elder daughter's health was poor (failure to thrive).

Mr A had lived on his own and worked locally since 1969. After his marriage, his family had remained with his parents in Bangladesh until his father's poor health had precipitated their move to England. They stayed in the small bedsitting-room which was part of Mr A's work contract. The accommodation was overcrowded; his wife became pregnant; and Mr A found himself in breach of his contract. He was dismissed and forced to leave the flat.

Weekly counselling enabled him to acknowledge and cope with the chaos and stress caused by his changed life circumstances, and his conflicting feelings about suddenly becoming a full-time husband and father with a family directly dependent on him. The social worker arranged temporary bed-and-breakfast accommodation for the family and discussed the case with the council's housing department and local housing association and, six months later, the family was adequately rehoused. The social worker also obtained financial assistance from a local charity which helped furnish and equip the new home. The third child was born shortly afterwards. Support was given to the family while they settled into their new neighbourhood where Mr A finally found suitable employment.

This work took one year. The social worker had strengthened the father in his role as caretaker of the family, dealing with both the emotional as well as practical aspects of resettlement and re-employment. In this way the family survived potential breakdown.

It is important to note that Mr A was Asian. Research indicates that black and ethnic minority groups feel more comfortable about accepting social-work help when it is recommended by their GP; in general they do not take full advantage of social services provisions. It would seem to be good strategy therefore, to locate a social worker in the general practice surgery to ensure that these people receive the help they need.

The social worker and health related social problems

The social worker is usually the member of the primary care team best equipped to deal with health-related social problems. Their special expertise includes knowledge of local resources. Patients will be referred on, as and when appropriate, and to appropriate agencies. The social worker has knowledge of child protection procedures; of relevant legislation; of sources of financial help. He or she usually has better working relationships with social services teams and housing departments and efficient networking skills. Without the involvement of a social worker, many cases such as Mr A's would not be allocated in the Social Services Department because they would not be considered to have high enough priority.

Patients referred to the social worker in general practice, are often already involved with other agencies: for example, the Social Services Department. Communication between GPs and the social services teams is frequently poor. The social worker can help strengthen these and similar relationships by promoting a greater understanding between the people involved. Working with the professional network is a vital and increasingly important role for GPs. For some patients, containment, and sometimes even staying alive, will depend upon the network of social services providing them with adequate support. This can happen only if the support is co-ordinated and not fragmented.

Patients who benefit most

Three distinct groups of patients benefit primarily from contact with a social work counsellor.

(i) *Elderly people and their carers.* The number of isolated, elderly, and frail elderly people is growing. Depression is common amongst the elderly and the GP may be their only contact for help. People who care for the elderly are also a very vulnerable group, often reaching the point of physical breakdown themselves. A social worker's efforts consisting of counselling, organising practical support and befriending, and running support groups for carers can be, when offered alongside GP medical services, the only help that many carers will accept.

(ii) *The mentally ill.* The number of mentally ill people in the country is increasing and the GP is usually the person first contacted for professional help. Many chronically ill patients are now found among the homeless; others less disabled who slip through community care networks will become so. To improve the quality of care for these people it is essential for the primary care team to work closely with other agencies and disciplines responsible for assisting these people in the community. The social worker in general practice is well placed to help.

(iii) *The under-5-year-olds.* The under-5s, and particularly the under-2s, place heavy demands on parents – particularly mothers. Regular social-work help achieved for example, by visiting mothers who are too depressed to come to the surgery, can provide vital support for a mother and thus help ensure both her and her baby's future mental health.

Conclusion

A psycho-therapeutically trained social work counsellor attached to a general practice can enhance the skills and the resources offered to the many patients presenting with health-related social problems. Their role is particularly significant for patients whose problems require co-operation between the general practice and several other support agencies within the community.

References

1. Corney R H. Social work in general practice. *J R Coll Gen Pract* 1985;**35**:291–292.

2. Bhaduri R. GP attached social work: a prescription for counselling. *Social Work Today* 1989;**21**(14):16–17.

Further reading

Balint E, Norell J S, editors. *Six minutes for the patient: interactions in general practice consultation.* London: Tavistock Publications, 1973.

Sanders K. *A matter of interest: clinical notes of a psychoanalyst in general practice.* Pitlochry: Clunie Press, 1986.

Address for contact

Mary Burke, The Surgery, 241 Westbourne Grove, LONDON W11 2SE

9. Counselling in General Practice

C   Options for Action: Person-centred counselling

CHRISTINE MANZI, Relate Counsellor in General Practice, North London

SUMMARY

A professionally trained counsellor employed as a regular member of the primary health care team can contribute significantly to the effective management of psychosomatic and emotional disorders and the effects of life stresses in that practice. The length, duration and severity of the problems, patient distress, and the often widespread effects of these difficulties are all beneficially affected by the use of person centred counselling. In the practice where I work, the inappropriate use of GP and hospital services by such patients has also decreased. Close co-operation between the counsellor, the patient's GP and the primary health care team is essential. More appropriate training and more frequent use of these services is advocated.

Background

For the past five years I have been employed as a counsellor in a large training general practice on the outskirts of London. The practice has nine doctors (partners) and a full complement of ancillary staff including a community psychiatric nurse (CPN) and social worker. I attend the surgery on two days each week, having previously spent many years working as a counsellor for the Marriage Guidance Council, now 'Relate'.

The problems encountered in the surgery are similar to those dealt with by Relate. The main difference is that the clients have chosen to visit their GP for help. And they are not at all surprised to be offered counselling rather than other forms of medical treatment. Most referrals come to the counsellor from the doctors; usually in the form of a short explanatory note. Appointments, made by me, are for 50 minutes on a regular weekly basis and usually for a period of six to eight weeks. Regular contact between the doctors and counsellor is an important part of the work. I attend practice meetings and we discuss referrals specifically each month.

Style: a personal approach

There is no one set style of practice. Professional skills and guidelines must be adapted to meet the needs of particular patients. This might be best illustrated via a case history as follows:

(i) Long-term intervention

'Joe' visited his GP because he was depressed (verbal presentation). The doctor told him he felt it would be helpful to see the counsellor and suggested that he made an appointment (negotiation). Joe agreed.

Information gathering

Joe appeared as a very presentable but dejected-looking young man of 36 (visual presentation) who was quite ready to tell me about his life (visual and verbal cues). He had a good job, but his girlfriend of nine-years-standing had recently left their joint home. All he wanted was for her to return. When he first came, he would say, 'There is nothing to tell you this week. She didn't come round.' I remember replying, 'You didn't exist this week then?'

Joe quite enjoyed his work and was doing well, but he had few friends or casual social acquaintances and was somewhat estranged from his family whom he saw only rarely. After work he went home and spoke to no one until he returned the next day. Weekends passed in a similar way. Occasionally, he drove to the coast and sat alone in his car watching people enjoying themselves on the beach. At night he slept in the car. Although he could well afford a hotel, booking in would involve speaking to someone. He was becoming increasingly isolated.

During the first weeks I found it very hard to keep awake during his sessions. An extreme heaviness overcame me (emotional cue). When I felt I had developed a sufficiently good relationship with him, I told him how I felt. 'That's funny,' he replied, 'Sometime ago I was treated for that feeling. It lasted for three years.' Indeed, his original problem had been extreme fatigue. He had been investigated at three different hospitals and eventually admitted for observation. Many treatments had been tried but all to no avail. The fatigue just 'went away'.

Action

Joe attended regularly. While I saw him weekly, his GP also saw him regularly but much less frequently. That contact between his doctor and myself was crucial – especially when I believed Joe to be suicidal. At one stage, he seemed to have totally given up, and an appointment with my supervisor provided the opportunity for beneficial discussion and support.

About four months after therapy began, without warning, and with absolutely no feeling in his voice (tonal cues), Joe told me of two instances of sexual abuse by a neighbour, experienced when he was 11-years-old. Although he felt he had become 'a bit more withdrawn' after this, he did not really feel that the events had affected him greatly. After discussing these issues for several weeks, I referred Joe to a therapeutic group, although I also continued to see him until he was established. This was to encourage him to say in the group what he could now say to me. It took him several weeks. As in his daily life, he was, at first, only an observer. However, once he was able to describe the abuse he began to realise its full impact on him. He began to get in touch with his feelings.

Outcome

As he made contacts within the group, Joe also began to make contacts in his personal life. He joined a squash club, began visiting the pub in the evenings, and met a new girlfriend. Much to his surprise, he realised people wanted to speak to him and he to them. Recently he wrote to tell me he was getting married. As counselling came to an end, Joe made another appointment with his GP to discuss the sexual abuse. He felt it would help the doctor understand what had been wrong with him all this time.

Comments

Joe demonstrates how much doctor and hospital time may be wasted through prolonged and repeated medical investigations. Had a counsellor been working in the surgery when he first presented, it is probable that Joe would have been referred directly to the counsellor after the initial investigations had been made and nothing found physically wrong.

(ii) Short-term interventions

Not all patients need such long courses of treatment. One woman, for example, referred because of panic attacks suffered on London's Underground Railway, needed to speak about an abortion she had arranged 20 years previously. She had never been able to talk about it to any one. The combination of menopause and the Kings Cross Station fire had reawakened feelings of what, to her, was her own disaster. Counselling sessions which lasted six weeks enabled her to recognise and accept the link between the emotional source and physical expression of her problem.

Conclusion

Counselling practised in the manner described does not prevent anxiety or depression in the patients referred. But it can decrease the length and severity (and thus the ill effects) of their distress: reduce the number of inappropriate demands made on GP and hospital services by these patients. Doctors who 'prescribe' counselling in preference to routine anti-depressants or tranquillisers should find this practice more effective, and professionally satisfying. To be effective, counsellors should be professionally trained and supported.

Further reading

McLeod J. *The work of counsellors in general practice*. London: Royal College of General Practitioners, 1988; occasional paper 37.

Irving J, Health V. *A guide for general practitioners*. Rugby (Warwickshire): British Association for Counselling: Counselling in Medical Settings Division, 1985.

Royal College of General Practitioners/British Association for Counselling. Information booklet on counselling in general practice. In press 1991.

Addresses for contact

(a) RELATE OFFICES

EAST: The Warden's House, 46 Crowndale Road, London NW1 1TR (Tel: 071 388 2665)

MIDLANDS: 'Sharlyn', Market Street, Penkridge, Staffs ST10 5DH (Tel: 078 571 5677)

NORTH EAST: 2nd Floor, 25 Micklegate, York YO1 1JH (Tel: 0904 644916)

NORTH WEST: 93 Bewsey Street, Warrington, Cheshire WA2 7JQ (Tel: 0925 572410)

SOUTH: 42 Holmesdale Road, Reigate, Surrey RH2 0BX (Tel: 0737 221511)

WEST: 16 Clare Street, Bristol BS1 1XY (Tel: 0272 214643)

(b) BRITISH ASSOCIATION FOR COUNSELLING

Counselling in Medical Settings Division, 37a Sheep Street, Rugby, Warwickshire CV21 3BX (Tel: 0788 578328)

(c) AUTHOR

Christine Manzi, Theobold Centre, 121 Theobold Street, Boreham Wood, Herts WD6 4PU.

9 Counselling in General Practice:

D Options for Action: The Nurse Practitioner/Counsellor

NICOLA MCFARLAND, Nurse Practitioner and Counsellor, West London

SUMMARY

The role of the nurse practitioner/counsellor in the primary care team is developing rapidly as the prevalence of emotional disorders and the benefits of early diagnosis and effective management are recognised. The nurse counsellor employed in general practice makes an important contribution to the initial recognition and care of such patients and is in an excellent position to prevent or minimise the effects of relapse or other problems. Doctors must recognise the need for and value of such posts and provide funds adequate for the purpose.

Background

A nurse practitioner (or practice nurse) with an extended role as counsellor, I work in a five-doctor general practice in Inner London which cares for 10,000 people. I have a Diploma in Counselling from the Lincoln Institute for Psychotherapy and currently attend a weekly seminar at the Parkside Clinic which was until recently, the Paddington Centre for Psychotherapy. The Clinic also gives me regular supervision for my patients. My interest in counselling derived from years in general practice which had convinced me of the value of having someone with the time and skills available to listen and help with problems which had social and psychological, as well as medical causes. Nine years ago, a senior partner in general practice encouraged me to help him cope with, in his words, 'the stream of human misery that pours through my surgery doors'.

Unlike many counsellors, I work as a full member of the medical team, having my own surgery and working from the medical notes. The doctors refer patients to me for counselling, but I will have already seen some of them previously for physical problems, or may indeed, have found counselling to be appropriate from my own observations made during a medical consultation. Practice nurses are in a very good position to detect distress in patients, many of whom find it less intimidating to talk to them than to the doctor. Referrals also come from hospitals or mental institutions seeking continued support for patients living in the community. Sometimes patients directly request counselling for themselves.

The nurse counsellor may also be asked to offer a second opinion. If the doctor is uncertain about the cause of a problem, I may be asked to perform a medical task while in fact assessing the mental state of a particular patient. The doctor and I then consult each other to determine the best line of treatment. There has certainly been an increase in the number of social problems seen in general practice. Perhaps we are taking over at least part of the role previously filled by the church or social services departments. Patients are given the opportunity to discuss family strife, economic problems and unsatisfied goals, anxiety, insecurity and sexual problems.

As a nurse, it is essential to observe and listen very carefully to each patient. Certain complaints or attitudes, or ways of presenting medical symptoms can indicate emotional problems. Not everyone who visits my surgery with a headache or sprained ankle is offered counselling, but it is unquestionable that many patients visiting the doctor for physical symptoms are masking an underlying emotional problem.

Counselling procedures

Patients in need of counselling are offered a half-hour appointment, usually in the afternoon when the surgery is less busy. This is a time for quiet assessment after which the patient may be offered four further appointments. At the end of this course the counsellor and patient together assess progress and determine further action. Options available are several and include: group or individual psychotherapy; behavioural therapy for obsessional neurosis; stress management, relaxation and therapeutic massage; breathing exercises and management of stress. Longer-term counselling at the surgery will be chosen for appropriate patients.

The average caseload is 12 regular patients a week. This number is doubled over a month by the attendance of regular patients who receive support counselling on a fortnightly or monthly basis. This programme means that the counsellor sees 70 patients a year which, on a four-day-week (including time taken for writing up case histories) represents a third of the total time of employment.

Patients suitable for counselling

Patients accepted for counselling, whatever their background, must be reasonably articulate and able to step back and observe themselves reflectively. They come from all age-groups, but may be grouped into five main categories:

(i) Rootless, solitary and lost people who do not seem to fit in with any group. Counselling support will allow them to function and give them effective relief while they learn to make more satisfactory personal relationships. I call this 'benign parenting'.
(ii) People suffering loss and separation: death, loss of love, loss of health, loss of the gratification of a particular stage in life, and regret about having to move on (eg, acceptance of retirement, children leaving home).
(iii) Loss of self-esteem and worth, either through failure at work or dissatisfaction from unhappy or abused childhoods.

(iv) People in crisis, where immediate help is required (eg, serious accident, sudden redundancy or suicide threat).

(v) 'Heart-sink patients'. These patients repeatedly present with trivial physical problems. Their aches and pains inevitably turn out to be emotional in origin. Just one session with the counsellor can make these patients feel much better and so reduce the many visits paid to the doctor.

Case histories

Polly

Polly, a 25-year-old woman came to the well woman clinic for a cervical smear. It soon transpired that she did not need a test as she had never had sexual intercourse. This admission released a flood of tears and fears about whether she was normal because she had never had a boyfriend. Questioning revealed that the underlying problem was related to family influences. Well-meaning but dominant and over-protective parents had stunted Polly's development as an adult. All the implications of growing up – making decisions and being independent – terrified her.

Polly was seen weekly for 18 months. It would have been inappropriate – indeed damaging – to break the trust established and refer her elsewhere, even though I would not normally undertake such long-term work. Polly was offered the chance to grow up in the safe confines of my surgery. She is learning to go from one phase of development to the next without having to shut the door on the last one. What had seemed like unbearable abandonment and loss have now become containable. She has developed self-confidence and esteem; can make her own decisions comfortably – even face disapproval and criticism. She is becoming a separate, adult person, able to make a happy and sexually fulfilled relationship.

'Mrs H'

A neat, ex-nurse in her 60s, Mrs H had visited her GP for several months complaining of post-viral symptoms: headaches, nausea and loss of energy and motivation. The doctor, sure that she was depressed, referred her to me. I, almost persuaded that she did have medical problems, could not tackle the emotional issues until more pathology tests had eliminated physical disease. The tests proved negative, but it took many weeks of counselling for me to penetrate the effective defense mechanisms which protected the core of her distress and enabled her painful feelings to be translated into physical problems. Gradually she was able to admit that her illness was something she could not cure by practical methods alone, or push aside with a 'stiff upper lip' approach.

We looked at her extreme anxieties together. She recognised that her obsession with time and punctuality was her way of maintaining control of her life and life situations. She learnt to let go of time and through behavioural treatment, learnt to be mildly slothful. Her anxiety evaporated as she accepted herself and allowed her expectations of herself to become more reasonable.

Relaxation tapes and exercises helped her recovery. The headaches and nausea disappeared, energy and motivation returned, and she was able to take part in her usual daily activities again. Apart from an arranged follow-up appointment, at which she looked well, relaxed and happy, she has not visited the surgery for nearly a year.

Comment

A general practice which includes a nurse counsellor on its staff is more effective and efficient. In the current climate, where there is a need to cut costs, provide better community care, and keep people away from hospitals, a nurse's 'normal' services are already in great demand. A nurse costs little, if anything, as many of the services he or she provides can be claimed for separately by the practice. In my practice, the presence of a counsellor has reduced the number of prescriptions written for benzodiazapines and antidepressants. It has also freed the doctors' time. My personal auditing attempts show that 90 per cent of patients I see for counselling do not concurrently visit the doctor. Their problems are contained and dealt with in our sessions.

GPs might believe that a nurse counsellor is unnecessary because they can provide the counselling themselves. This may be so, provided that the doctor has learnt the necessary skills and can organise the practice to avoid unnecessarily long waiting times for patients with more physical problems. A nurse/counsellor can provide the support and expertise needed to avoid such unnecessary, but common, disruption.

Conclusion

There is a growing need for counselling services able to deal with the many social and emotional problems seen in general practice. Counselling services should be an integral part of modern general practice. Appointments should be offered to the patient without stigma being attached, and without undue delay. The emphasis should be on short-term work which involves a high degree of commitment between the patient and the trained counsellor.

Address for contact

Nicola McFarland, The Medical Centre, 2 Garway Road, London W2 4NH

10 Liaison in Primary Care: Early Detection of Difficulties

A. Preventing Child Neglect

KEITH BESWICK and PAULINE RICHARDSON, Didcot Health Centre, Oxfordshire

SUMMARY

The general practice-based Didcot Group started in October 1975 as a response to the perceived need of parents having problems coping with their children. The Group drew on local, central and voluntary resources for funding and manpower. Reconstituted as the Friday Group in 1984, it has maintained its original aim to prevent rather than treat child abuse, and its success may be attributed largely to the close liaison established between trained professionals in the Social Services and primary care team.

1. The Didcot Child Abuse Prevention Project

Keith Beswick

Background

Mention of Didcot, a town set in South Oxfordshire, probably brings to mind sleepy villages and a rural economy. That picture, true before World War II, ended irrevocably with the building of the Harwell Laboratory for the Atomic Energy Research Establishment, the Didcot power station, the M4 and M40 motorways and the British Rail Intercity Express network. Starting practice there in 1972, I was appalled by the lack of help available to the many young mothers and their children in the area – especially when they had trouble coping with everyday domestic responsibilities and problems.

My first case of child abuse presented with petechial marks of asphyxiation. The child's family was 'Army': the Army solved the problem by moving them elsewhere. My partners then encouraged me to find out more about this newly-emerging condition.

Sharing the load: preparing a team

Margaret Lynch, an expert in the subject at the Park Hospital, Oxford, challenged us at a lunchtime gathering of local health professionals to do something practical to help these mothers and their young offspring. A survey of the 9,000 patients then cared for by the practice primary health care team revealed that the parenting of some 30 children (from 22 families) was giving cause for concern. Sexual abuse was not seriously considered 15 years ago: if it had been, the task confronting us might have seemed too daunting and the project might never have got underway.

A research grant paid by Action Research for the Crippled Child enabled us to employ a research social worker, Jackie Roberts, from the Park Hospital for the first six months of the project. The first task undertaken was to identify the *skills and support needed* by health professionals working in such an emotionally-charged minefield. Among those highlighted were:

How to

(i) come to terms with a personal sense of failure
(ii) stop identifying with a family
(iii) learn to live with a sense of helplessness having to accept the situation globally and for the family
(iv) implement action within limited resources
(v) deal with anxieties about working with a potentially lethal situation
(vi) cope with the hope that 'If I bury my head in the sand, it will all go away'.

Defining local resources

Then, as now, money was tight. We had to clearly determine, and differentiate, 'real' from 'apparent' resource options. Table 10.1 shows that this essential exercise, although somewhat discouraging, was not devoid of humour – or benefit. As a result, planning and management programmes were more soundly based: the Didcot Project began unencumbered by rose-coloured expectations!

The Didcot group begins work

Conditions which contribute to child neglect or abuse are rarely quickly or easily eliminated. A group approach was therefore adopted to tackle them in

Table 10.1 Defining local resources

Resource	
As offered (theory)	**As practised (reality)**
24-hour life line	'I am not very helpful when woken at 2 am!'
Therapeutic relationship	'Whatever that means – I am sure we all (already) offer it.'
Child care – provision of	'Social Services still have no money!'
Practical family help	'Have no fear. Supergran is here!'
Referral to other (specialist) agencies	'I (the GP) have the distinct feeling I am about to become an 'other' (specialist) agency! I already deal with: asthma, cervical cytology, diabetes mellitus, geriatrics, immunisation, paediatrics, minor surgery, practice management, employment, law, computing etc, etc. . .'

Didcot as it could save much valuable GP consultation time (compared to one-to-one interviews) while giving patients more time and involving them actively in their own problem-solving. Eight women were invited to join a group, held for two hours each week in the health centre, while their children attended a separate meeting in the centre's child guidance playroom. This latter group was led by a trained occupational play therapist aided by two non-qualified assistants and student volunteers from the local secondary school.

Jackie Roberts and I acted as co-therapists for the first six months in the mothers' group; then Jackie was replaced by a local social worker. A male presence proved very useful. Excessive 'male-bashing' was moderated – though much of it was justified – and enabled the women to gain insight into how they sometimes provoked aggression in their partners and how they might avoid this. We had found it very difficult, when setting up the project, to involve fathers.

Funding

The research grant covered only the first six months of operation. We were able to qualify for a health promotion clinic fee, but initially, I spent more time raising money than working in the group. Today, the group is run as a service provided by the Social Services and the Community Unit.

Progress and problems

Mothers often have a low self esteem, and once lost, self respect can take years to recover. People with little self respect isolate themselves. Relationships between partners and friends break down; the confidence needed to seek out and develop social supports evaporates. They have unrealistic expectations of themselves, their children, their immediate and 'extended' families, and of the professional support services, including primary care.

Children attending the group had problems separating from their mothers. They were too insecure to leave them. The need for a trained play/occupational therapist was quickly demonstrated and she helped overcome many difficulties and episodes of disruptive acting-out behaviour which continued until the child learnt new skills and felt secure within the group. *Frozen watchfulness* was a common occurrence of as much concern as acting-out. Children would not join in with the others until they developed a sense of belonging and felt secure enough to act as/be, a child. Several successes gave impetus to the work. One little boy for example, discharged from hospital with the label of 'grossly delayed development and failure to thrive', is now a normal, gangling, six-foot teenager.

Strategies

The group was initially on trial – with both professional colleagues and participants. We all had a lot to learn. Confidence and trust had to be earned and established between members themselves and between them and the professional therapists. The women, individually and as a group, wanted to know 'How safe is it to come?'; 'How much can I safely reveal about myself?'; What will X think if I reveal my *real* self?'; 'Do they *really* care about me?'.

Trust was only slowly established as a group identity emerged. Members began to reveal personal truths; share and then redefine problems more realistically; bolster self respect by being able to give as well as receive help – with even very intimate problems. The group itself – perhaps not surprisingly – was sometimes viewed with suspicion or even feared by professional colleagues not directly involved with its work. One senior doctor in a neighbouring practice forbade his patients to consult me about child abuse. Yet, it was still acceptable for me to give their dental anaesthetics! Such resistance, still apparent in Didcot seven years after the group began, can make it very difficult for women and their families to find the help they need in time to prevent physical abuse or further loss of confidence and self respect. In 1984, I gave up my work as co-therapist in the group to become a trainer in general practice.

Professional benefits

Working with the group provided me with an insight into life and relationships not available from one-to-one consultations. I learnt to give more than lip service to the value of support provided by colleagues. The time and effort required to establish and then maintain the group paid dividends in the long term. It is very important to consider these factors in general practice because it does take time to provide more than the basic services.

Conclusion

The advantage of having a resource like the Friday Group as it became, is that it is possible to ask parents if they are coping with their children in a way which allows them to say 'no' without suffering further 'loss of face' or recrimination. The group also offers them the opportunity to contribute to the resolution of their own problems while sharing confidences with and giving help to mothers in similar situations. For the GP, it offers a resource which frees him or her from the time needed for one-to-one consultation over a considerable period of time. It does not however, isolate the patient from the practitioner, and it is effective only provided that the practitioner is able to sense and diagnose the problem and refer patients appropriately.

2. Under new management: The Friday Group

Pauline Richardson

After Keith Beswick retired as co-therapist in 1982, the Didcot Group was reconstituted as the Friday Group. No longer attached to general practice, it was modified to fit current demands and indeed, is regularly revised to ensure that it remains in touch with the needs of local families. This has been helped by establishing a drop-in centre in the town for mothers which is staffed by voluntary workers. The Group meets there weekly during term time, and is a combined health visitor, social worker, and family aide scheme for mothers with children under five years, who are having difficulty coping. Their problems remain many and varied; all cause distress. A mother with two or more children under five might for example, become suicidal after the break-up of her marriage; another, a happily married woman, but unhappy mother, although not clinically ill, can unless she receives help from the group, place heavy demands on the health visitor or GP.

The mothers' group

Health visitors, social workers and GPs refer mothers to the group which is led jointly by a social worker and a health visitor. A closed group, it follows specified ground rules which address basic procedures such as disclosure and confidentiality. Confidentiality is breached only if actual child abuse occurs, or if a child is considered to be in danger. The mother is then kept fully informed of any action taken.

The group now provides a well-established, well respected and safe, adult environment where mothers can discuss their difficulties as *they* see them – free from the judgement of family and friends, or the distractions caused by demanding children. Identification of the problem behind the symptoms takes time. Time passed in the company of interested, trusted listeners is needed to help participants discern or disclose the problems causing their symptoms; to recognise areas of stress and personal need; to set priorities for action. All may be addressed by the group together, or individually with a group leader.

Family problems are frequently complex. Team meetings are necessary to consider the many aspects of such problems and determine an effective strategy. Information newly received from the family aide, health visitor, social worker, and other members of the primary care team who know the mother concerned is collated and considered immediately after the Friday gathering. Recommendations are then made which can be put into practice at once, thus providing essential support and hopefully, preventing further deterioration – incuding possible child abuse.

The crêche

An important subsidiary to the mothers' group is the crêche run by two family aides and a voluntary helper. Knowing that their children are being well cared for enables the mothers to concentrate on the business at hand in the group. For children, the crêche provides a secure stimulating environment, where they benefit directly by having fun while developing skills and positive relationships with attentive adults as well as children of a similar age. To ensure maximum effect, the adult:child ratio is kept at 3:10. The family aide's observations of the children's appearance and behaviour provide essential information necessary to accurately assess progress and plan further management of the families' difficulties.

Conclusion

The Friday Group in Didcot is a facility which provides an effective means for the detection and prevention of possible child neglect. It does this successfully because of the close liaison established between trained professionals in the social services and the primary health care team. The strength of this professional co-operation, and its ability to encourage support from local voluntary organisations is an essential ingredient for success.

Address for contact

Dr Keith Beswick and Mrs Pauline Richardson, Didcot Health Centre, Asbury Medical Centre, Britwell Road, Didcot, Oxfordshire OX11 7JH.

10 Liaison between Providers of Primary Care: Early Detection of Difficulties

B Predicting Postnatal Depression

DEBORAH SHARP, Senior Lecturer in General Practice, United Medical and Dental Schools of Guys and St Thomas's Hospitals, London

SUMMARY

This paper describes an explanatory model for postnatal depression which supports work first published by Brown and Harris in 1978. It suggests that postnatal depression occurs in women who possess certain vulnerability factors and for whom the pregnancy acts as a provoking factor. These predictive factors can be detected most readily during pregnancy and the puerperium by the general practitioner and members of the primary care team. Early intervention, aided by support from relevant professional colleagues and services, the woman's family and friends, and local self-help groups can effectively prevent or modify the illness. Essential elements for success are professional awareness of the prevalence of postnatal depression; close liaison between members of the primary care team; and the provision of information about psychological reactions to childbirth for pregnant women, new mothers and – where possible – their partners.

Background

This section examines the prediction of postnatal depression in the context of liaison between providers of primary care. In keeping with the conference theme – the prevention of depression and anxiety – it discusses prediction as a tool for prevention and uses the term 'postnatal' depression quite specifically within the spectrum of emotional disorders which occur after childbirth. It does not cover:

(i) *puerperal psychosis* – the severe illness which affects only 1–2 women per 1,000 soon after delivery and usually requires admission to hospital (preferably to a specialised mother and baby unit); or

(ii) *the 'baby blues'* – the transient dysphoria which affects up to 50 per cent of women in the first post-partum week and usually remits spontaneously.

Childbirth is an experience of great psychological significance and for many women will be their most important life event. Society would have us believe that it is a universally happy event. But research shows that the months

Figure 10.1 *Temporal relationship between psychiatric admission and childbirth: (a) all admissions; (b) psychosis admissions*

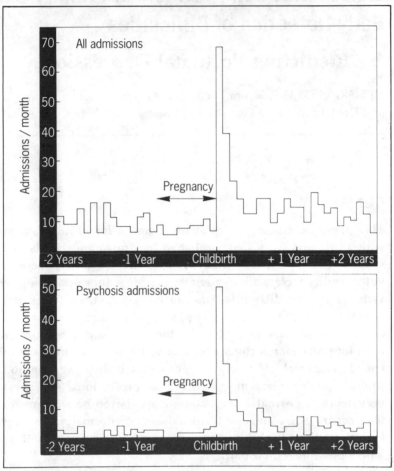

Reproduced with kind permission from Kendall R E, Chalmers J C, Platz C. *Br J Psychiatry* 1987 **150**: 662

surrounding the birth pose the greatest lifetime risks for women of developing a mental illness[1] (see Figure 10.1).

Postnatal depression is just one of the psychological disorders associated with childbirth, but from a public health perspective, it is probably the most important. Evidence suggests that it affects at least 10–15 per cent of women in the first postnatal year, usually beginning in the first three months[2,3,4]. This depression can mark the start of a chronic, relapsing illness, or a relatively short-lived episode which will never recur. In either case, the consequences for the woman herself, both at home and at work, for her partner and the quality of their relationship, and for her family and friends, can be irrevocable. Adverse effects on the mother/infant relationship and subsequent child behaviour and development can be profound[5,6].

What exactly is postnatal depression?

Postnatal depression can certainly be included in the hidden psychiatric morbidity which GPs are being exhorted to uncover. The wide variation in symptomatology makes it difficult to diagnose, especially since many women are unaware that their symptoms are due to depression – particularly if somatic problems predominate. The clinical features of postnatal depression are essentially those of a neurotic depression, with anxiety and irritability accompanying depressed mood. Tearfulness and fatigue contribute to a feeling of general inadequacy. Poor concentration, loss of appetite and insomnia are common, as too are vague physical symptoms, such as headache, backache and vaginal discharge for which no cause can be found. Loss of libido is often marked and can further damage an already strained marital relationship. A few women have obsessional thoughts about harming their baby, and for an even smaller minority, the level of misery is so great that suicide is contemplated.

Clinical symptoms and signs

A mother suffering from postnatal depression may present in many ways, but two very common examples are:

(i) *The unhappy, tearful and exhausted mother* who frequently visits the surgery – usually on account of her children – is familiar to everyone in primary care. Hopefully, most GPs recognising this woman's distress, would enquire generally about *her* health and more specifically, about *her* mood and how *she* was feeling – regardless of whether the consultation was for herself or for one of her children.

(ii) *Masked depression*. This mother, who rarely consults, comes in smiling, always looks immaculate, and only describes physical symptoms. Suddenly, her guard is down. Behind the smile is a woman overwhelmingly concerned with appearing to be the perfect mother and wife. In reality, there are tears and torture: worries about feelings for the baby; concern about her imminent return to work; loss of libido and its effects on the marriage; problems keeping up with the housework and other domestic duties. Generally, she is not coping as well as she would like.

The message to be learned is: *Any new mother can develop postnatal depression!*

Is postnatal depression a distinct syndrome?

Although the existence of puerperal psychosis has been known for well over 100 years, it is only in the last 20 or so, that postnatal depression has been recognised as a separate diagnostic entity requiring treatment. However, its acceptance is not universal. Neither puerperal psychosis nor postnatal depression appears in the International Classification of Diseases 9 (ICD–9). Furthermore, there have always been those professionals – both medical and non-medical – who have denied its existence, expecting mothers with young babies to 'stop grumbling'; 'get on and cope', regardless of the enormous difficulties they might experience.

At the other end of the spectrum, the Women's Movement has helped bring postnatal depression before the public eye. It has alerted women to the possibility of emotional causes for their physical symptoms and has increased the sensitivity of health care professionals to their psychological needs.

Two recent reports by Cooper (1988)[7] and O'Hara (1990)[8], which question whether there is an increased incidence of depression after childbirth, have provoked considerable controversy. However, these studies were not carried out in general practice and they used somewhat inappropriate outcome measures of psychiatric disorder.

Current evidence favours the existence of postnatal depression as a distinct syndrome seen mainly by GPs and other primary care professionals. As such, it does not always meet the requirements imposed by rigid psychiatric diagnostic criteria for classification as 'typical' (ie, major) depression. However, this level of depression can still be extremely distressing and disabling.

Past research

Many of the original studies of postnatal depression were conducted by GPs who observed an increased incidence of depression amongst postnatal patients in their care. Tony Ryle, a GP in North London in the late 1950s, assessed the incidence of psychiatric disorders associated with childbirth[9]; David Tod studied 700 women in an urban practice in the late 1950s–60s in an attempt to define psychological disorders which arose during pregnancy and the first postnatal year[10]. In 1970, Blair and a group of GPs in Devon, who had a special interest in psychiatry, looked for predictors of postnatal depression in their antenatal patients[11]. One of the group, Playfair, later mounted a multi-centre study[12], involving 64 GPs. This aimed to identify symptoms, signs, and other conditions which, when present during the antenatal and perinatal periods, indicated that depression was likely to occur after the birth. One criticism of these early studies in general practice is the lack of definition of the term 'depression' and the inherent difficulty in comparing their results. In 1986, Ancill and his colleagues successfully used a computer-delivered questionnaire to screen women for symptoms of antenatal and postnatal depression when they attended antenatal clinics and postnatal check-ups in general practice[13].

Most of the research over the last 20 years has come from mental health professionals working in hospital antenatal clinics and on postnatal wards. Brice Pitt, a psychiatrist, prompted much of this interest by publishing his description of 'atypical depression following childbirth' in 1968[14]. But as noted above, postnatal depression is very definitely a general practice disorder – *typical* of the sorts of the depression seen every day by GPs in their surgeries. Psychiatrists rarely see it in their hospital practice, and as stated, it does not conform to the rigid diagnostic criteria set for major depression. This is why Pitt called the depression in his study, 'atypical'.

Determining risk factors: prospective research

If postnatal depression exists, what is its epidemiology? Some consensus exists between the studies undertaken by mental health professionals to determine likely risk factors, but translation of these predictors into a programme for prevention in primary care is hindered by the bias in these studies towards hospital rather than general practice populations. To rectify this bias, a prospective, longitudinal study of childbirth-related emotional disorders in primary care was undertaken between 1986 and 1988, which examined prevalence, natural history and predictive factors.

Methodology

The study involved two general practices in South London: one in the inner city, and one, with a large population of young families, in a new town on the outskirts of the city. Two hundred pregnant women were followed up from early pregnancy until the end of the first postnatal year. Just under half were pregnant with their first child. They were predominantly white British women (78 per cent); married (60 per cent); and working class (86 per cent). Their average age was 26 years, half had not planned the pregnancy (45 per cent), and roughly one third (37 per cent) had previously seen a GP for an emotional problem.

Self-report questionnaires and standardised psychiatric interviews, administered at each woman's home on up to four occasions, provided the data for analysis. Information about emotional wellbeing – *specifically*: anxiety and depression, personality, life events, attitudes towards pregnancy and the baby, the quality of the marital relationship, and past medical history – as well as basic demographic data was collected.

The Clinical Interview Schedule (CIS)[15], a standard psychiatric assessment developed for use in community surveys, was used to determine the presence or absence of psychiatric disorder at each assessment. Significant disorder ('a case') was recorded when a participant scored more than one on the Overall Severity Rating (OSR) of the CIS. The vast majority of these disorders were classifiable as ICD9 neurotic depressions or depressive adjustment reactions. The proportion of cases found at each of the assessments (12–14 weeks pregnant, 36 weeks pregnant, 3 months and 12 months postnatal) was similar – around 25 per cent – with a drop to 19 per cent at the one-year-postnatal interview. The period prevalence for pregnancy (ie, the percentage of women who were assessed as 'a case' at least once during pregnancy) was 38 per cent and for the postnatal year, 33 per cent.

Major risk factors in postnatal depression

Table 10.2 demonstrates the most important factors found to be associated with psychiatric disorder at each assessment (determined by Chi-square analysis).

In early pregnancy and at 36-weeks-gestation, the risk factors were very similar, but the strength of the associations differed. The importance of socioeconomic factors and the strength of the marital relationship are emphasised.

At 3-months-postnatal, the most interesting finding was the lack of association between psychiatric disorder and 'hard' obstetric factors such as gestation, hours in labour, type of delivery, episiotomy, or the level of pain experienced. 'Baby-related factors' associated with depression included delay in holding the baby, having the 'blues', insufficient help after the baby was born, and

Table 10.2 *Risk Factors for Concurrent Psychiatric Disorder during Pregnancy and the First Postnatal Year*

	Early Pregnancy	Late Pregnancy	3/12PN	1YRPN
Poor Social Support	***	***	***	***
Poor Marital Relationship	***	***	***	***
Past Psychiatric History	***1	*	***	
Financial Problems	***	***	**	
Unplanned Pregnancy	***2	*	*	
Adverse life events in (previous 6 mths)	***	***	4	***
Obstetric History	**	***		
Unemployment	*	*		
Housing Problems	*	*	*	
Worry about Labour	*	*		
Coping Poorly with Baby			**	
Delay in Holding Baby			*	
Post Partum Blues			*	
Wanting to Work/Being at Home				***
Problems with Baby				*3
Number of HV Visits				*

*>0.05 ** P>0.01 *** P>0.0001
1=particularly with history of postnatal depression
2=particularly if termination considered
3=other than ill health
4=not enquired for

generally not coping well with the infant. Pre-existing social problems were still important.

At one-year-postnatal, fewer significant associations with depression were found. The only 'baby-related' factor reported was problems due to behaviour (eg, feeding, crying and sleeping) – but not ill-health. The number of home visits by the health visitor was also relevant, but it was unclear whether these were influenced by problems with the baby or the mother's health. Marital problems, poor social support and financial problems were still associated with increased likelihood of psychiatric disorder. Wanting to work but not being able to for some reason, and thus being left at home all day, posed a significant risk.

Comment

This study uncovered a large amount of depression in women seen during their pregnancy and in the first postnatal year. The rate is probably a true reflection of the level of distress and misery because it is confirmed by the correlation of the results obtained in psychiatric interview with those obtained from self-report questionnaires. One of the strongest predictors for postnatal depression was a past psychiatric history – recorded either before or during the pregnancy. Figure 10.2 shows that depression occurring during pregnancy greatly increases the likelihood of depression in the first postnatal year.

Figure 10.2 *Prior psychiatric problems in 200 women with (and without) postnatal depression in general practice; London 1988.*

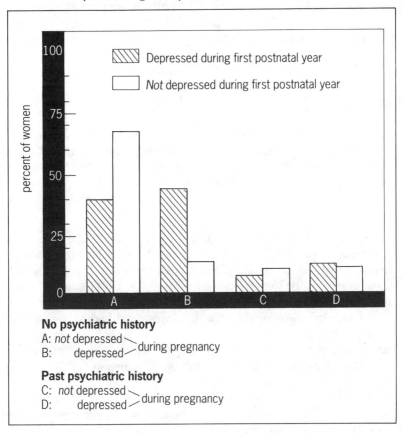

It is interesting to note that there was no association between depression at any time in the study with the basic demographic variables – marital status, social class, ethnic origin, education or parity – and by the end of the postnatal year, an unplanned pregnancy no longer seemed to be a significant risk factor. These findings generally agree with those first published by Brown and Harris in 1978, in *Social Origins of Depression*[16].

Predictors as a tool in prevention

The predictors found here reflect information which GPs usually have in their records, but which is not always recognised as being of particular relevance to pregnancy. They cover areas well within the GP's remit. Antenatal care programmes in the UK offer the primary care team the opportunity to prevent postnatal depression by discerning the presence of risk factors and tailoring the subsequent care to meet each woman's needs. Closer attention to the psychological processes accompanying pregnancy and childbirth will enhance a mother's overall enjoyment of this important event. Regular contact with the primary care team, both before and especially in the early period after the birth, when the mother first returns home, will allow the detection of mood changes and social difficulties much earlier and so, facilitate preventive action. Close, consistent contact is essential for women thought to be at risk of postnatal depression.

Practising prevention

As the results show, psychosocial factors did predict postnatal depression, but factors related to delivery did not. This indicates that closer attention to the pregnant woman and new mother's psychosocial environment will provide a better opportunity to practice prevention. The resources available are considerable (see Figure 10.3), but they must be used effectively.

The importance of liaison

The GP is the lynch-pin in the primary care team, having the advantage of closer and often more prolonged contact with the pregnant woman and new mother than do other health professionals. However, close liaison between all members of the support network identified in Figure 10.3 is essential for the delivery of effective care. Practical examples of the benefits of working in this way include:

(i) *Obstetricians* having better access to information about their patients' psychosocial problems. This would help them in making decisions about management: eg, about admitting women for bed-rest or perhaps allowing them to stay a little longer after delivery.

(ii) *Hospital midwives* could hand out self-report questionnaires at antenatal clinics to help screen for risk factors. Women with high scores could then be referred to

(iii) *a liaison psychiatrist* (or psychologist) within the obstetric service who could then maintain contact with both the woman and her GP – if necessary, into the postnatal period[17].

(iv) *Community midwives* could undertake some of their hospital counterparts' duties. They are well placed to discuss concerns about previous obstetric problems and the coming delivery.

(v) *Health visitors* could be put in contact with women early in their pregnancy in order to develop trust and to detect potential causes and early signs of depression.

Figure 10.3 *Professional and personal support available for women during pregnancy and the first postnatal year.*

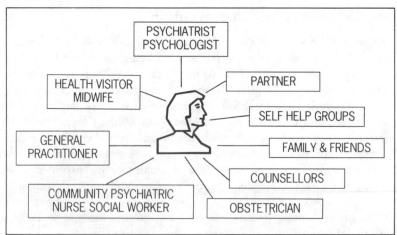

(vi) *Community psychiatric nurses* can provide the special support needed by women showing signs of mental illness. A study done in South London showed that support groups, led by a psychologist or social worker for women thought to be at risk of postnatal depression, helped reduce the incidence of depression found at six months after the birth[18].

(vii) *Social workers* can help relieve financial pressures by ensuring that women and their families receive appropriate and maximum social benefits.

(viii) *Trained counsellors* (from various backgrounds) can help women who have specific problems: eg, with their marriage, or with drug or alcohol dependence.

(ix) *Husbands and partners* who attend antenatal clinics and evening classes in parentcraft, gain a greater appreciation of the psychological, as well as the physical, changes that their wives are experiencing. They also learn how the baby's arrival is likely to influence established partnership and life-style patterns.

(x) *Family and friends* can be encouraged to help with other children and domestic chores – rather than be entertained in return for admiring the baby!

The GP working within this network thus has both a direct and a co-ordinating role in ante- and postnatal care. The focus of each consultation will vary – from clinical examination to pastoral-style enquiry and counselling. Listening to a woman's worries early in her pregnancy will help establish the quality of relationship needed to detect risk factors or early signs of depression, and where necessary, arrange appropriate referral. The six-week postnatal follow-up offers GPs the opportunity to ask 'how things are at home' and to assess the mother's mood – as well as take her blood pressure and a cervical smear. Some doctors also routinely give out self-report questionnaires, such as the 10-item Edinburgh Postnatal Depression Scale, which seem to offer a reliable method of detecting clinically-significant depression[19]. Others reserve them for women who seem depressed (ie, as a confirmatory measure) or at risk of depression.

Secondary prevention

Once depression is confirmed, secondary prevention measures come into play: early detection offers the best hope of effective treatment. It may be appropriate for the GP to prescribe anti-depressants. Alternatively, other resources are considerable. Health visitors, for example, have achieved success by involving mothers in non-directive counselling sessions[20]; referral to an appropriately-trained counsellor, psychologist, or psychiatrist might be advisable; and specialised self-help groups, such as the *Association for Postnatal Illness* or voluntary organisations such as *Home-Start* which provide trained helpers in the home (see Chapter 13A) can also give support. A joint consultation between a family doctor, and a husband and wife might be all that is needed to bring to light some of the causes for the wife's distress, and by so doing, to help the husband understand and help resolve the problem(s).

Conclusion

Postnatal depression can affect any mother in the year following the birth of her child. Risk factors which may be used to predict such depression have been identified. They are not surprising – poor social support, adverse life events, an unplanned pregnancy, a poor marriage, financial difficulties, housing problems and a past psychiatric history. The pregnancy is the straw that breaks the camel's back! GPs and members of the primary care team can use these risk factors to practice prevention and avoid depression. However, for a successful outcome, it is necessary to:

(i) dispel the myth that postnatal depression is an uncommon disorder which invariably requires referral to a psychiatrist;

(ii) give pregnant women (and their partners) information about normal and abnormal reactions to childbirth, so that they can ask for help when necessary; and

(iii) most important, ensure that the primary care team can predict which women are the most vulnerable, so that preventive measures can be instituted early. Close liaison between members of the primary care team is essential for a successful outcome.

References

1. Kendall RE, Chalmers JC, Platz C. Epidemiology of puerperal psychoses. *Br J Psychiatry* 1987; **150**: 662–673.

2. Cox J L, Connor Y, Kendell R E. Prospective study of psychiatric disorders of childbirth. *Br J Psychiatry* 1982; **146**: 111–117.

3. Elliott S A, Rugg A J, Watson J P, Brough D I. Mood changes during pregnancy and after the birth of a child. *Br J Clin Psychol* 1983; **22**: 295–308.

4. Kumar R, Robson K. A prospective study of emotional disorders in childbearing women. *Br J Psychiatry* 1984; **144**: 35–47.

5. Cogill S R, Caplan H L, Alexandra H, Robson K M, Kumar R. Impact of maternal postnatal depression on cognitive development of young children. *BMJ* 1986; **292**: 1165–1167.

6. Caplan H L, Cogill S R, Alexandra H, Robson K M, Katz R, Kumar R. Maternal postnatal depression and the emotional development of the child. *Br J Psychiatry* 1989; **154**: 818–822.

7. Cooper P J, Campbell E A, Day A, Kennerley H, Bond A. Non-psychotic psychiatric disorders after childbirth. A prospective study of prevalence, incidence, course and nature. *Br J Psychiatry* 1988; **152**: 799–806.

8. O'Hara M W, Zeloski E M, Philipp L H, Wright E J. Controlled perspective of postpartum mood disorders: comparison of childbearing and non-childbearing women. *J Abnormal Psychology* 1990; **99**: 3–15.

9. Ryle A. The psychological disturbances associated with 345 pregnancies in 137 women. *Journal Mental Science* 1961; **107**: 279–86

10. Tod E D M. Puerperal depression: a prospective epidemiological study. *Lancet* 1964; **ii**: 1264–1266.

11. Blair R A, Gilmore J S, Playfair H R, Tisdall M W, O'Shea M W. Puerperal depression: a study of predictive factors. *J R Coll Gen Pract* 1970; **19**: 22–25.

12. Playfair H R, Gowers J I. Depression following childbirth – a search for predictive signs. *J R Coll Gen Pract* 1981; **31**: 201–208.

13. Ancill R, Hilton S, Carr T, Tooley M, McKenzie A. Screening for antenatal and postnatal depressive symptoms in general practice using a microcomputer-delivered questionnaire. *J R Coll Gen Pract* 1986; **36**: 276–279.

14. Pitt B. Atypical depression following childbirth. Br J Psychiatry 1968; **114**: 1325–1335.

15. Goldberg D P, Cooper B, Eastwood M, Kedward H B, Shepherd M. A standardized psychiatric interview for use in community surveys. *British Journal of Preventive Social Medicine* 1970; **24**: 18–23.

16. Brown G W, Harris T. *Social origins of depression*. London: Tavistock, 1978.

17. Appelby L, Fox H, Shaw M, Kumar R. The psychiatrist in the obstetric unit: establishing a liaison service. *Br J Psychiatry* 1989; **154**: 510–515.

18. Elliott S, Sanjack M, Leverton T J. *Parents groups in pregnancy – a preventive intervention for postnatal depression*. In: Gottlieb B H, editor. Marshalling social support. London: Sage Publications, 1988.

19. Cox J L, Holden J M, Sagovsky R. Detection of postnatal depression. Development of the 10 item Edinburgh Postnatal Depression Scale. *Br J Psychiatry* 1987; **150**: 782–786.

20. Holden J M, Sagovsky R, Cox J L. Counselling in a general practice setting: controlled study of health visitor intervention in treatment of postnatal depression. *BMJ* 1989; **298**: 223–226.

Further reading

General

Motherhood and Mental Illness, Vol 1. ed: Brockington IF, Kumar R. London: Academic Press, 1982.

Motherhood and Mental Illness, Vol 2. ed: Kumar R, Brockington IF. London: Wright, 1988.

Questionnaires and tests

Snaith RP, Bridge G W K, Hamilton M. The Leeds Scale for self-assessment of anxiety and depression. *Br J Psychiatry* 1976; **128**: 156–165.

Goldberg D. *The detection of psychiatric illness by questionnaire*. London: Oxford University Press, 1972.

Barnett B E W, Hanna B, Parker G. Life event scales for obstetric groups. *J Psychosom Res* 1983; **27**: 313–320.

Kumar R, Robson K M, Smith A M R. Development of a self-administered questionnaire to measure maternal adjustment and maternal attitudes during pregnancy and after delivery. *J Psychosom Res* 1984b; **28**: 43–51.

Address for contact

Dr Deborah Sharp, Department of General Practice, United Medical and Dental Schools of Guys and St Thomas's Hospital, 80 Kennington Road, London SE11 6SP.

11 Liaison between Primary and Secondary Care Teams towards Early Intervention

A A general approach

GERALDINE STRATHDEE, Consultant Psychiatrist, Maudsley hospital

SUMMARY

This chapter explores the subject of how general practitioners and mental health specialists should liaise in the assessment, treatment and prevention of mental illness.

Close liaison between general practitioners, primary care teams, and specialist psychiatric services ensures the best use of available personnel and resources. The different strategies by which such co-operation is being developed are described.

Introduction

The subject of how general practitioners and mental health specialists should liaise in the assessment, treatment and prevention of mental health disorders has long been of interest to health care planners and clinicians alike[1,2]. Particular concerns include: has the extent of psychiatric morbidity in primary care increased as a result of the policies of deinstitutionalism and community based psychiatric treatments? What should be the relative roles of primary care and psychiatric teams in the identification and treatment of patients with neurotic conditions such as depression and anxiety and those with psychotic disorders? How can the organisation of the mental health teams be improved to facilitate liaison and improve the quality of care? What practical strategies can GPs undertake to enhance their treatment of illness and enable them to practice prevention?

Psychiatric morbidity and the balance of care

Well known studies, in general practice[3] indicate that between one-fifth and one-quarter of all consultations to the average general practitioner are patients with mental health problems, and that the vast majority of these are managed in the primary care sector without recourse to specialist care. General practice consultations for identified psychiatric disorder outnumber psychiatric out-patient attendances by roughly 10:1 and psychiatric admissions by roughly 100:1[4]. More recently, however, in his analysis of the Third National Morbidity Statistics, Smeeton[5] demonstrated that general practitioners have become increasingly reluctant to use psychiatric diagnostic terms for psychosocial problems. This trend, if widespread, would have significant implications for studying the workloads of general practitioners, counsellors, the specialist mental health services and the manner in which they liaise.

The development of community care facilities has not kept up with deinstitutionalisation policies[6]. General practitioners have, therefore, an increasing burden of responsibility for severely mentally ill people in the community[7] as well as their long standing role in relation to detection and treatment of depression and anxiety. This includes the physical and psychiatric care of those discharged from psychiatric institutions, the homeless, patients treated in their homes who might previously have been admitted to in-patient units or respite facilities[8]. Many such patients seek help from general practitioners[9] and they may be reluctant to re-attend a psychiatric hospital[10,11].

The Roles of Primary and Secondary Care Teams

What then should be the relative roles of primary care and psychiatric teams in the identification and treatment of patients with psychological disorders? Many models of interaction have been proposed including three outlined by Williams & Clare[12]. The first of these was the 'replacement model' which referred to the notion that psychiatrists should replace the GP as 'the doctor of first contact'. The American community mental health centre movement exemplifies this model but its validity for the bulk of patients with psychological disorder in this country is questionable. Furthermore, it runs counter to the policy of the World Health Organisation[1] which proposes that the primary care physician should be the 'cornerstone of community psychiatry'.

The second model has been described as the 'increased throughput model' which suggested that an increase in the number of psychiatrists would provide the GP with the ability to refer more patients with psychological morbidity. To some extent this model has been tried and found wanting, in that between 1970 and 1975, there was a 28 per cent increase in consultant staff and a 35 per cent increase in the number of junior staff in the UK, with no resultant increase in either the number or rate of new patient referrals. The third model, named the 'liaison-attachment model' was based on the conclusion drawn by Shepherd[13], in his original work in which he states 'that administrative and medical logic alike suggest that the cardinal requirement for the improvement of mental health services in this country is not a large proliferation of the mental health services, but rather a strengthening of the family doctor in his therapeutic role'.

Currently, new prominence has been given to finding the most appropriate and effective relationship between psychiatric and primary care teams. The debate over the relative merits of the separatist or integrated approaches described above continues unabated. In the current development of community psychiatric services there has been a trend among psychiatrists to separate the planning and resource needs of those with neurotic conditions such as depression and anxiety from those with chronic and psychotic disorders. Many in the secondary care services would argue that, with the limited financial and manpower resources available, the only valid work of psychiatric teams or professionals such as CPNs is with the latter group. This faction would claim that the care of those with depression and anxiety is most appropriately undertaken by the primary care team including counsellors, attached psychologists or others funded by GPs themselves.

An alternative view is that this separatist approach fails to take account of the continuing reality that, for the majority of patients, whatever the nature of their disorder, primary care forms the point of first contact and often acts as the central base from which other care is obtained[14]. From this perspective, what is needed is an integrated approach in which the secondary care team has an important role to play in assisting primary care teams to develop the skills needed to support patients with psychiatric difficulties, and to learn more themselves about the nature and extent of psychiatric problems seen in general practice. Opportunities for such mutual learning occurs at many different points of service contact and the optimal format for such liaison has been the subject of study in a new wave of research. Methodologies have concentrated on auditing the needs of district GPs and in the evaluation of the models of liaison clinics undertaken by psychiatrists working in primary care settings.

What general practitioners want from liaison with the psychiatric services

Three audit studies have focused on the determining the needs of GPs in relation to the development of district community psychiatric services[14,15,16]. The first of these took place in the context of an initiative to develop community based services in Camberwell. The district's 154 general practitioners were consulted to ascertain the attributes of the existing crisis, consultation and in-patient services which they found most helpful in meeting the needs of their patients and to propose apposite future initiatives. This study has been described in detail elsewhere[14] and only a brief summary of the pertinent liaison issues will be presented here.

Crisis Services

Crisis intervention in Camberwell was provided: on a full 24 hour basis by a crisis intervention clinic; and by the domiciliary consultation service. Table 11.1 summarises the attributes of crisis intervention found most useful by GPs. *Access to an immediate specialist opinion* was regarded as essential, a finding confirmed by other research[15].

Table 11.1 *General Practitioner Requirements from Crisis Services*

Provision of an immediate opinion
Personal contact with senior psychiatrist
Home assessment
Outreach service
Crisis service for parasuicide assessment
Rapid access to a MHA assessment
Training in the Mental Health Act

Nationally, domiciliary consultation is probably the most common form of crisis intervention available since the inception of the National Health Service in 1948, but is a very expensive resource, and costs the NHS 20 million pounds a year. Psychiatry comes second only to geriatric medicine in the number of such consultations requested[17]. The Camberwell GPs *preferred the home setting* of the domicilliary assessment, which enabled the psychiatrist to gain insight into the social and physical environment of the patient. They also found the *personal contact with a senior psychiatrist* helpful, in contrast to what one commentator regarded as the inevitable consequence of teaching hospital practice, 'you send the patient to hospital and they almost invariably see a Senior House Officer with less experience than I have'.

Domicilliary assessment was originally set up to provide a joint consultation between a consultant and a general practitioner for the specific purpose of making an assessment of the patient and formulating an agreed management plan. It was intended to take place only if the patient was, for medical reasons unable to come to hospital[18]. However, the practice of joint visits is fast disappearing. In a retrospective six month analysis of a district's domiciliary consultations one survey has shown that only one-third were appropriate referrals and none were undertaken jointly with the referring GPs[19]. Valuable opportunities for communication and mutual education are thus lost.

In general, the audit studies show that GPs are unhappy with their level of training in the use of the Mental Health Act and value rapid assessment by the specialist. In the development of the new community services two innovations were proposed: an outreach team which would visit patients at home and an assessment facility for patients who had taken overdoses or attempted suicide. Some of the GPs have emphasised that any outreach service should be available on a 24 hour basis[16].

Outpatient Services

The early research demonstrated that of all patients with mental health problems presenting to primary care, only 5 per cent were referred on for a specialist opinion[13]. Referral practices vary enormously between general practitioners for a complex mixture of personal, professional, social and clinical reasons[20]. Perhaps it is not therefore surprising that the success of the specialist services in addressing such a diversity of need has been limited[20]. General practitioner dissatisfaction with traditional hospital outpatient services is well documented in relation to long waiting lists, inadequate and tardy communications, tendency to create chronic careers for attenders and a lack of clear guidelines on management[21,22].

Almost two decades on, GPs in the Camberwell Survey were just as critical as their predecessors had been. Table 11.2 gives details of the strategies suggested by GPs for improving the quality of outpatient services. Many of these relate to communication between referrers and specialists and include: a longer management section in letters; clear statement of the objectives of the treatment, current and future levels of medication, future plans in terms of psycho-

Table 11.2 *General Practitioner Requirements from Outpatient Services*

Rapid assessment
Shorter referral-appointment interval
Better communications
Clear management guidelines
Statement of objectives of treatment
Predicted response, complications and side-effects
6 monthly review plans for chronic patients
Clearly stated role of GP and specialist in treatment
Clarification of prescribing responsibilities
Information booklets of therapies available

therapies and counselling and six-monthly written reviews for patients with long term disorders.

For patients in whom it had been possible to identify pre-morbid symptoms of relapse, GPs wanted to be alerted to the pattern of symptoms and signs, and to be advised about suitable interventions, including medication, stress-reducing strategies, and psychotherapy. Many of the general practitioners asked for descriptions of behaviour therapies, cognitive therapies, counselling and the various psychotherapies to which they had not been exposed during their training. What was also wanted was a named liaison person who could advise on appropriateness of referral in departments offering these therapies. Access to information booklets on medication and other therapies, effects, side-effects and expected outcomes was recommended, much like those produced by MIND and mentioned in Chapter 8.

Attachments of mental health professionals to primary care

Since the 1970s there has been a growing trend for psychiatrists to establish formal attachments to primary care settings. A survey in 1984[23] found that almost 20 per cent of English and Welsh psychiatrists spent at least one session per week working in this way. A similar survey in Scotland[24] found that almost half the Scottish psychiatrists had regular contact with primary care teams. A range of models of liaison attachment have been described[23,25]. These involve various degrees of interaction between the referring GP and the attached specialist. At its most informal, the psychiatrist meets the practice GPs for a *'lunchtime meeting'*. Without setting an agenda, management issues concerning individual patients or aspects of the doctor-patient relationship can be raised and discussed.

This approach is formalised in the *'consultation'* model where the referrer presents specific cases to the psychiatrist, who advises on diagnosis and management, but does not see the patient and the treatment is undertaken by the primary care team.

The most commonly applied format is the *'shifted outpatient'* model where the secondary care team moves the hospital outpatient list to the primary care site.

This facilitates communication and joint assessment and treatment. Having agreed a management plan, the GP assumes the primary role in treatment, seeking the advice of the specialist as appropaite.

At its most sophisticated, this may evolve into the *'liaison-attachment team'* model[26]. Here a close working relationship is fostered between the multi-disciplinary teams of both the primary care and mental health services. This has advantages in terms of training and resource allocation. As the primary care team, with psychiatric support, becomes more familiar and confident in the assessment and management of psychiatric disorders, so the need for psychiatric input becomes less intense. This frees the psychiatric team to form links with new practices.

For certain groups of patients who are reluctant to return to the 'stigmatising' outpatient clinic, for example women, the homeless, and young people with schizophrenia, primary care psychiatric clinics may be the only way to provide care and practice prevention[10,27].

Psychologists, nurse therapists, CPNs, social workers, counsellors have also formed links with primary care teams, (see chapter 9).

Our Camberwell GPs regarded CPNs as a valuable resource and wanted to have direct access both to them and to psychologists. However, they were less enthusiastic about the notion of having one of these disciplines undertake regular sessions in the surgery. Yet both in this survey, and others[25,26] practices which have 'attached psychiatrists' have reported benefits including; improved liaison and continuity of care, the facility to make joint assessments and undertake treatments, the ability to obtain advice on patients at an early stage in the development of illness or relapse, the development of new skills and techniques, an increase in knowledge of psychiatric disorders and treatments, a decrease in admission rates and more multi-disciplinary teamwork.

The Role of the General Practitioner

Much of the previous text has concentrated on general practitioners referring patients to the mental health agencies. A pertinent issue however, is the extent to which general practitioners have either the necessary interest, time, skills, training and resources to undertake psychological treatment and practice prevention themselves. Concern has been expressed that general practitioners are being deskilled by more automatic, prompt and earlier referral away to the numerous attached professionals and counsellors. However, it is clear that GPs value the improved level of knowledge gained in their close contact with 'attached' psychiatrists. The Camberwell GPs specifically requested training in behavioural techniques and cognitive therapy using a format of skills, learning workshops and open distance learning.

Making Use of the Consultation

Even without such sophisticated ventures, GPs may wish to consider the range of clinical and organisational strategies proposed below aimed at facilitating

Table 11.3 Issues for Psychiatrists and GPs Working Together

Development of good practice protocols
Pre-referral work and use of the waiting time
Use of screening questionnaires
Adaptation of new treatment techniques to GP
Education and support of families
Participation In Care-coordination
Participation in joint audit

---

prevention and early intervention (Table 11.3). Making good use of the consultation is not only a preoccupation of GPs. It is also crucial for psychiatrists. In many districts in Great Britain there is only one trained consultant psychiatrist for sectors of between 35,000 and 65,000 population, and outpatient consultation times may be similar to the 12 minutes available for those with psychological dysfunction in primary care.

One of the principle advantages GPs report of behavioural-cognitive therapy is the effective use of time available. In it GPs will recognise the common-sense, practical approach needed in their discipline. France & Robson[28] have produced an excellent text which aims 'not to turn every GP into a behaviour therapist but rather to enable him/her to adapt the effective techniques of behavioural-cognitive therapies to the time constraints of their own work'.

Making Use of Wasted Time

One of the most frustrating times for patients and their doctors is the interval between consultations or between the referral to a specialist and receiving an appointment. In our local health centre, this hiatus led both mental health and primary care teams to initiate strategies to use the time more productively. These included the keeping of diaries in order to monitor diet, drug or alcohol intake, the time and duration of anxiety attacks, the monitoring of aggressive episodes in relation to stimulating and other life-events, and the completing of a life-chart of medical, social, psychiatric and other concurrent events.

Better Assessment of the Mental State

The ability of general practitioners to detect psychiatric morbidity varies greatly. Although they have the advantage of being uniquely placed among medical disciplines in that they more frequently live in the communities where they work, this can also have disadvantages for interview. General practitioners have often commented on the difficulties of asking certain questions of a psychological nature to people who are not only patients but may also be neighbours or professionals in their own right, ie the dentist, the hairdresser, or the childminder. Posing the question 'Do you have suicidal thoughts'? can alter the nature of a relationship quite fundamentally. Two initiatives are useful here: The use of video-feedback techniques to effect improvement in interview techniques (see chapter 5) and the modelling effect of joint assessments in primary care clinics when the generalist observes how to ask 'embarrassing' questions and respond appropriately when positive responses are elicited.

Deborah Sharp (see chapter 14) has discussed using the Edinburgh Questionnaire to detect women with post-partum problems. Other standardised questionnaires may be helpful in the detection and assessment of disorder and their application may focus the consultation more efficiently. Examples include the CAGE, to identify people with alcohol problems, the Beck, which monitors change in patients with depression and the GHQ, which detects non-psychotic ill-health.

Caring for patients with longterm mental health disorders

Patients with long-term mental health disorders have a broad spectrum of requirements which includes their need for physical care, recognition and treatment of relapse, crisis intervention and the education and support of families and carers. Up to 40 per cent of patients with severe long term psychiatric morbidity have concurrent physical problems[29] and their treatment may play a vital role in the rehabilitation process. As one of my patients commented, 'before I had my corns seen to, they said I wasn't *motivated* to go to the day centre.' General practitioners, with their comprehensive knowledge of the social and medical history of their patients, are also probably in the best position to pick up early signs of a relapse in the patient.

Care Co-ordination

The NHS and Community Care Act dictates that local health authorities and social services draw up jointly agreed community care plans based on assessment of the multiple needs of patients with long-term mental health problems. As the traditional co-ordinators of care, GPs have much to offer in the implementation of systems of case-management which should follow this policy. As a pragmatic unresourced initiative our sector team in Greenwich has evolved a care-co-ordination approach. In this, the client and all individuals involved in his or her care (including GPs, social workers, CPNs, psychiatrists, voluntary organisations, and housing departments), meet to develop an *Individual Patient Plan* which identifies problems, sets three-six monthly objectives and clearly defines individual responsibilities in meeting patient needs. This approach requires evaluation but our early analysis indicates that it decreases unplanned consultations to psychiatrists, to GPs and to emergency departments, improves the level of patient functioning, facilitates early detection of relapse, enables more rapid and accurate communication and has greater patient and professional satisfaction.

Joint Audit

Audit is a relatively recent activity which presents new opportunities for joint collaboration. In both the Camberwell study[14] and that by Ferguson[15], GPs had the opportunities to influence the structure and working of their local service. It is disappointing that in the latter study, which examined a service before, and four years after, the introduction of community-focused, multi-disciplinary team, only 40 per cent of the primary care doctors participated in the second stage. For the future it may be that the creation of purchaser/provider contracts will both facilitate and force the two disciplines to work together to develop good practice proformas which will improve standards in the assessment, treatment and prevention of mental health disorders.

Conclusion

For the future we would do well to follow the advice of Horder[30] who asserts that through clinical work, organisation and education, the alliance between psychiatrists and GPs will give patients the benefit of the marriage between expertise on one side and comprehensiveness and continuity on the other.

References

1. World Health Organisation. *Psychiatry and primary medical care*: WHO Regional Office for Europe, 1973

2. Paykel E, Mangen S, Griffith J, Burns T. Community psychiatric nursing for neurotic patients: a controlled trial. *Br J Psychiatry* 1982, **140**: 573–81.

3. Goldberg D P, Blackwell B. Psychiatric illness in general practice: a detailed study using a new method of case identification. *BMJ* 1970, **ii**: 439–443.

4. Jenkins R, Shepherd M. *Mental illness in general practice*. In Mental Illness: Changes and Trends. (Ed) P Bean. Chichester: Wiley, 1983.

5. Smeeton N C. Episodes in mental illness in general practice: results from the Third Morbidity Survey. *Health Trends* 1989, **2**, 63.

6. Griffiths R. *Community Care: an Agenda for Action*. London: HMSO, 1988

7. Kendrick A, Sibbald B, Burns T, Freeling P. Role of general practitioners in care of long term mentally ill patients. *BMJ* 1991, **302**: 508–511.

8. Thornicroft G, Bebbington P. Deinstitutionalisation: from hospital closure to service development. *Br J Psychiatry* 1988, **155**: 739–753.

9. Johnstone E C, Owens D G C, Gold A, Crow T J, MacMillan J F. Schizophrenic patients discharged from hospital – a follow-up study. *Br J Psychiatry* 1984, **145**: 586–590.

10. Tyrer P. The 'hive' system: a model for a psychiatric service. *Br J Psychiatry* 1985, **146**: 571–575.

11. Brown R, Strathdee G, Christie-Brown J, Robinson P. A Comparison of Referrals to Primary Care and Hospital Outpatient Clinics. *Br J Psychiatry* 1988, **153**: 168–173.

12. Williams P, Clare A W. Changing patterns of psychiatric care. *BMJ* 1981, **282**: 375–377.

13. Shepherd M, Cooper B, Brown A, Kalton G. *Psychiatric illness in general practice.* Oxford University Press, 1966

14. Strathdee G. Psychiatrists in primary care: the general practitioner viewpoint. *Family Practice* 1988, **5**: 111–115.

15. Ferguson B. Psychiatric clinics in general practice—An asset for primary care. *Health Trends* 1987, **19**: 22–3.

16. Stansfeld S. Attitudes to developments in community psychiatry among general practitioners. *Psychiatric Bulletin* 1991, (in press).

17. Fry J, Sandler G. Domiciliary consultations: some facts and questions. *BMJ* 1988, **297**: 337–338.

18. Littlejohns P. Domiciliary consultations – who benefits? *J R Coll Gen Pract* 1986, **36**: 313–315.

19. Sutherby K, Srinath S, Strathdee G. The Domiciliary Consultation Service: outdated anachronism or essential part of community psychiatric outreach? Unpublished research report, 1991

20. Kaeser A C, Cooper B. The psychiatric out-patient, the general practitioner and the out-patient clinic; an operational study: a review. *Psychol Med* 1971, **1**: 312–25.

21. Williams P, Wallace B R. Psychiatrists and general practitioners – do they communicate? *BMJ* 1974, **1**: 505–7.

22. Todd J W Wasted resources: referral to hospital. Lancet 1984, **2**: 1089.

23. Strathdee G, Williams P. A survey of psychiatrists in primary care: the silent growth of a new service. *J R Coll GenPrac* 1984, **34**: 615–618.

24. Pullen I M, Yellowlees A. Is communication improving between general practitioners and psychiatrists? *BMJ* 1985, **290**, 31–33.

25. Mitchell A R K. Psychiatrists in primary health care settings. *B J Psychiatry* 1985, **147**: 371–370.

26. Creed F, Marks B. Liaison psychiatry in general practice: a comparison of the liaison-attachment scheme and the shifted outpatient clinic models. *J R Coll Gen Pract* 1989, **39**: 514–517.

27. Joseph P, Bridgewater J A, Ramsden S S, El Kabir D J. A psychiatric clinic for the single homeless in a primary care setting in inner London. *Psychiatric Bulletin*. 1990, **14**: 270–1.

28. France R, Robson M. *Behaviour therapy in primary care*. London: Croom Helm, 1986
29. Brugha T S, Wing J K, Smith B L. Physical health of the long-term mentally ill in the community. Is there unmet need? *B J Psychiatry* 1989, **155**: 777–82.
30. Horder J. Working with general practitioners. *Br J Psychiatry* 1988, **153**: 513–521.

Address for contact

Dr Geraldine Strathdee, Consultant Psychiatrist, Maudsley Hospital, Denmark Hill, London SE5 8AF.

11 Liaison between Primary and Secondary Care Teams toward Early Intervention

B Assertive Help for Inner City Distress

STEVE ONYETT, Team work project manager, Research and Development for Psychiatry

SUMMARY

This paper argues for early intervention in urban mental distress through assertive and autonomous case-work within a managed-team framework in collaboration with general practice, and presents the Early Intervention Service (EIS), an Inner-London community mental health team, as an example. Details of the rationale for early intervention and the positive outcomes for users of the EIS (particularly those diagnosed as schizophrenic) will appear in a later paper in this series[1]. The present discussion focuses on management and practice within the EIS and all descriptive data are based upon a review undertaken after two years of operation.

Background: the EIS

The EIS comprises the usual multidisciplinary mix of community mental health nursing, social work, psychology, psychiatry and occupational therapy personnel. It currently has 10 members with one person in a co-ordinator role. The EIS is based in office accommodation which makes it absolutely necessary to see users in their own homes, and serves a highly ethnically and socially diverse population of around 120,000 in a four-mile patch of Inner London.

The aims of the service are to:

(i) maintain users in as normal a social context as possible, by intervening early to minimise disturbance and distress and avoid unnecessary admission;
(ii) rapidly deliver problem-orientated multidisciplinary clinical interventions in 'ordinary' environments;
(iii) provide an accessible mental health service by working jointly with other agencies;
(iv) continually monitor and evaluate the service provided.

The target client group are people aged between 16 and 64 years, who are experiencing a level of distress or disorder which, in normal circumstances, may, in the long or the short term, lead to hospital admission. A controlled evaluation has shown that the EIS provided significantly better service-user satisfaction and shorter hospital stays when compared with standard hospital-based care for people presenting as emergencies[2]. A very positive response was also received from referrers to the service[3]. Every individual who referred someone to the EIS in its first year was asked to indicate agreement with hypothetical statements about the EIS on a five-point scale (from 'strongly agree' to 'strongly disagree'). Half the statements provided were construed in favour of the EIS and half against.

The significance of deviations from the mid point for each statement (ie, neutral verdict) were tested using two-tailed Wilcoxon signed rank tests. All significant findings were in favour of the EIS. Table 11.4 shows the questions in order of statistical significance. The EIS policy of joint work was the most highly valued feature, and there was a very strong feeling among the sample that the EIS should become a permanent part of local services. This subsequently occurred. The fact that the service was accessible and community-based was also valued. Least approval was given for the appropriateness of the service for typical clients seen by the referrer. This suggests that considerable selection took place before referrals were made.

Pointers towards positive outcomes

The following points highlight important aspects of the work of the EIS.

Open referral

A service should be efficient in targeting its client group. This can be considered in terms of *horizontal* and *vertical target efficiency*[4].

Horizontal efficiency refers to the need for a service to be maximally accessible to any person who might make use of it. This incudes issues of physical

Table 11.4 *Referrer ratings of service aspects of Early Intervention Service*

Statement topics	Z	Significance	Percentage responders in favour of EIS
Multi-agency working	−6.74	$p<0.0001$	98
Whether service should become permanent	−6.62	$p<0.0001$	95
Working away from hospital	−6.53	$p<0.0001$	97
Ease of referral	−6.22	$p<0.0001$	91
Suitability for people from ethnic minorities	−5.52	$p<0.0001$	69
Speed of response to referrals	−5.29	$p<0.0001$	77
Communication from the EIS	−5.03	$p<0.0001$	79
Use for finding other forms of support	−4.83	$p<0.0001$	64
Suitability for homeless people	−4.5	$p<0.0001$	60
Use in helping with practical problems	−3.96	$p<0.0001$	50
Perceived satisfaction of users	−3.58	$p<0.0003$	56
Use for people with severe mental health problems	−2.63	$p<0.0085$	53
Use for people with long term problems	−1.05	not significant	47
Relevance to referrers clients	−0.22	not significant	41

Table 11.5 *Sources of referral to the Early Intervention Service*

Referrer	Count	Per cent
Self	33	6.5
General practitioner	178	35.3
Community psychiatric nurse	6	1.2
Area social worker	44	8.7
Health visitor	22	4.4
Psychiatrist	42	8.3
Unit social worker	53	10.5
Accident and emergency departmet	12	2.4
General hospital	2	.4
Psychotherapy	7	1.4
Police	1	.2
Probation service	12	2.4
Residential agency	23	4.6
Voluntary	19	3.8
Friend or neighbour	9	1.8
Other	41	8.1
Total	504	100.0

accessibility, publicity, routes of referral, and perceptions of the service as culturally relevant and non-stigmatising. The EIS invested a lot of energy into publicity and into personally visiting key people to clarify the aims of the Service and its methods. This high profile has been maintained by working jointly with other agencies. Totally open referral yielded the range of referrers shown in Table 11.5. GPs continue to make most referrals. In common with other approaches to open referral[5], this did not lead to a flood of inappropriate requests: 80 per cent of the people referred were allocated to a case manager following assessment. The others were (i) not seen for assessment despite repeated attempts: (ii) immediately admitted to hospital; or (iii) returned to the referrer with advice on more appropriate referral. The proportion of self referrals to the EIS is also increasing as people re-refer themselves.

Eligibility criteria based upon need

Vertical target efficiency refers to the necessity of gatekeeping. In order to meaningfully evaluate the work of a service and manage its workload, there has to be a system for prioritising referrals. Too often, this is based upon gross criteria which do not reflect current need, such as diagnosis, route of referral or history of service usage (eg, use of in-patient services). Social factors are far superior to diagnosis or clinical factors in predicting the onset, course and outcome of mental distress and the ways people make use of services[6].

The EIS uses three criteria to determine priority for the form of assertive, community-based interventions on offer: *severity and urgency, mental state and the need for community-based assessment*. Each represents a continuum, with more specific inclusion and exclusion criteria at either end. Although they are in descending order of importance, a person could compensate for a low score on one continuum with a high score on another. Thus, although the ideal candidate would be someone needing to be seen urgently in their home environment because of the effects of delusions or hallucinations, the criteria do not exclude people who would not be diagnosed as having a major mental disorder, but who, nonetheless, are experiencing severe distress.

According to referrers, around 27 per cent of referrals had to be seen within 48 hours, and a further 20 per cent within the next week. Of the people taken on for case management, 16 per cent were perceived as experiencing a stress reaction – usually following some life event such as separation, abuse, eviction, unemployment or bereavement. A further 34 per cent were diagnosed as having some form of anxiety or depression, and 21 per cent with schizophrenia. Over half were single, 60 per cent female, 42 per cent unemployed, and 14 per cent Afro-caribbean. About 63 per cent lived in rented accommodation, and around 20 per cent were homeless, living in bed and breakfast accommodation or resettlement units. Approximately a third had significant medical problems such as circulatory or heart disorder, or undernourishment.

Team work

Using the above criteria, the EIS endeavours to reach the most difficult-to-serve people living in the community. The demands of case-work with users and carers, and the need to maintain a clear and up-to-date picture of existing local resources require an accessible pool of knowledge, skills and experience. Two clinical review meetings per week provide the forum for the exchange of essential information.

Effective team working is achieved through the assumption of a case management role by team members within a clear organisational framework. The team co-ordinator role helped maintain clarity regarding responsibilities and lines of accountability, and provided a mechanism for the resolution of conflict[7].

Effective inter-agency working

Joint working is essential in order to prevent the discontinuity and fragmentation so characteristic of mental health services. At referral, all referrers are asked if they are willing to perform a joint assessment with members of the team. GPs and social workers particularly valued this option. The aim is to complement the work of other agencies involved rather than usurp it. In the case of GPs, joint assessment and subsequent work in the familiar non-stigmatising environment of the surgery led to good attendance on the part of service users, and high levels of collaboration and communication between the GP and the EIS worker. With this in mind, before an assessment is made, it is established whether the individual referred is already involved with other agencies. If a hospital-based team is involved, their permission is sought before intervening. The only exception is when the referral comes from a GP, because they take primary responsibility for the welfare of their patients. Whatever the circumstances, if others are involved, they are invited to participate. In practice, around 44 per cent of referrals are assessed jointly with other agencies.

Table 11.6 *Site of clinical work, Early Intervention Service (EIS)*

Site	Assessment		Subsequent Contact	
	Count	Per cent	Count	Per cent
Home	225	51.6	197	51.2
Hostel	32	7.3	26	6.8
Hotel	60	13.8	42	10.9
General practice	56	12.8	54	14.0
Hospital	28	6.4	20	5.2
Day centre	10	2.3	22	5.7
Other	25	5.7	24	6.2
Total	436	100.0	385	100.0

Assertive case management

Joint working is also promoted by delivering services to where the user spends most of his or her time. Thus, the EIS was able to work jointly with GPs in their own surgeries, key workers employed in hostels and health visitors visiting bed-and-breakfast families. Table 11.6 indicates the site of assessment and subsequent contact with service users.

Most importantly, taking services to users maximises the involvement of unpaid carers in assessment and subsequent work. Considerable evidence, both here and abroad, indicates improved outcomes for service users when assertive approaches are compared with more reactive approaches[8,9,10].

There is little evidence that this message is being heard in Britain. We have known for a long time that most mental health problems are addressed in primary care[11], yet disproportionate resources continue to be poured into hospitals[12] rather than the places where people prefer to be assisted[13].

Planning around the needs of individuals

Maintaining a continuous relationship between two people: a service user and a case manager, serves as a vehicle for individually-tailored provision. Assessment of needs and strengths, and service planning, delivery and review, around individual service users, is the core of this approach. Where individual service plans contain information about met and, more importantly, unmet need, they can be meaningfully aggregated to inform needs assessment at locality level, and thus, a process of contract development between purchasers and providers.

What of the future?

If services for people with severe and long-term mental health problems can be more clearly located within primary care or community-based services, this can only be to the good – particularly if it avoids the potentially-damaging effects of hospital admissions[14]. However, there is a danger that aspects of the new community care policies may impede continuous and co-ordinated care. The health and social care divide provides an opportunity for purchasers to attempt to divest themselves of costs as they haggle over responsibilities for providing care. It is crucial that health authorities, local authorities and Family

Health Services Authorities (FHSAs) get together at the earliest stages to collaborate on sharing information and jointly commissioning services. Teams such as the EIS provide a jointly-commissioned point of access, for service users and referrers, where the health and social care divide remains behind the scene. Multi-agency boards of senior managers charged with managing ring-fenced budgets allocated for the work of case-management teams, are a logical corollary of these arrangements. They would be able to receive information on met and unmet need, in order to inform the development of contracts.

The American literature gives little grounds for optimism regarding the mixed economy of care[15], indicating monopolistic providers offering a reduced quality of services, with higher staff turnover and severe discontinuity of care. Broad and co-ordinated purchase of service systems will be absolutely critical to avoid this. Also, since no demonstration programmes have yet claimed to be able to eliminate the need for some form of asylum care altogether, the flexible use of such services could usefully come within the purview of the (multi-agency) managing board or its parent organisations.

Conclusion

Managed teams of skilled workers undertaking the tasks of case management offer us the possibility of co-ordinated, continuous and cost-efficient care for people with severe and long-term mental health problems. Working assertively with users and carers in their own environments in collaboration with their GPs may also promote their autonomy and the maintenance or development of supportive social networks. If purchasers are to fully exploit this opportunity for tertiary prevention they must:

(i) give priority in resource allocation to services for people most difficult to serve;
(ii) shift resources away from hospital care towards services which work with service users and carers in context;
(iii) be clear about the allocation of responsibility for collecting and using information on outcomes for service users; and
(iv) use this information to inform the future resourcing of provider agencies.

New developments, such as the introduction of FHSAs into the purchasing arena, the mental illness specific grant, the care programming approach and community care plans may all promote these objectives. Key stakeholders (including users and carers) now need to work jointly at all levels to exploit these opportunities in the interests of high quality services.

References

1. Tyrer P. *Schizpphrenia: early detection, early intervention.* In 'The Primary Care of Schizophrenia. Jenkins R, Field V, Young R. (Eds) London: HMSO, 1992

2. Merson S, Tyrer P, Onyett S, Lynch S, Lack S. A controlled evaluation of early intervention in psychiatric emergencies. Unpublished manuscript, available from the author.

3. Onyett S, Tyrer P, Connolly J, et al. The Early Intervention Service: the first eighteen months of an Inner London demonstration project. *Psychiatric Bulletin* 1990;**14**:267–269.

4. Challis D, Davies B. *Case management in community care: an evaluated experiment in the home care of the elderly*. Aldershot: Gower, 1986.

5. Hagan T. *Accessible and acceptable services*. In: P Huxley et al, eds Effective community mental health services. Aldershot: Avebury/Gower, 1990.

6. Huxley P et al. *Effective community mental health services*. Aldershot: Avebury/Gower, 1990.

7. Onyett S, et al. *Case management in mental health*. London: Chapman & Hall, 1992.

8. Hoult J. Community care of the acutely mentally ill. *Br J Psychiatry* 1986;**149**:137–144.

9. Bond G R, Miller L D, Krumweid R D, Ward R S. Assertive case management in three CMHCs: a controlled study. *Hosp Community Psychiatry* 1988;**39**:411–418.

10. Modrcin M, Rapp C A, Poertner J. The evaluation of case management services with the chronically mentally ill. *Evaluation and Program Planning* 1988;**11**:307–314.

11. Goldberg D P, Huxley P. *Mental illness in the community: the pathway to psychiatric care*. London: Tavistock, 1980.

12. House of Commons. Social Services Committee. *Community care: services for people with a mental handicap and mental illness: eleventh report from the Social Services Committee*. Session 1989–90. London: HMSO, 1990. Chairman: Frank Field. (HC 664).

13. Personal Social Services Research Unit. *Care in the community newsletter*. Canterbury: University of Kent, May 1990.

14. Lipton F R, Cohen C I, Fischer E, Katz S E. Schizophrenia: a network crisis. *Schizophr Bull* 1981;**7**:144–151.

15. Schlesinger M, Dowart R A, Pulice R T. Competitive bidding and states purchase of services: the case of mental health care in Massachusetts. *Journal of Policy Analysis and Management* 1986;**5**:245–263.

Address for contact

Steve Onyett, Teamwork project manager, Research and Development for Psychiatry, 134–138 Borough High Street, London SE1 1LB.

12 Health Information

A A Health Education Library in General Practice

CLARE PACE, Practice Librarian,
Dib Lane Surgery, Leeds

SUMMARY

A plethora of health-related information has filled the popular press, media and commercial outlets with a confusing avalanche of programmes, publications, videos and audio cassettes. To help patients differentiate 'fact from fiction', or reinforce advice given by their family doctor during a standard 10-minute consultation, a health education library was set up nine years ago in a general practice waiting room. A review of this service shows benefits for both staff and patients. Mental health and child care were two of the most popular topics studied and access to the library has encouraged users to adopt healthier lifestyles.

A patients' library in general practice

One way of helping patients benefit from the useful elements of the surfeit of 'popular' information on health topics is to make a selection of it available in the surgery through a patients' library. Such a library was set up at Dib Lane Surgery in Leeds, nearly nine years ago, just at the beginning of the 'explosion' in health-related literature. Two partners in the practice, Arnold Zermansky and Chris Varnavides found themselves increasingly prescribing reading material for their patients, as well as more conventional medicines. Both believed that, if their patients were going to be able to help manage their own illnesses, or indeed prevent illness, they would need to reinforce the information given them in the average 10-minute consultation. One way to do this was to send the patients home with a book to read and perhaps discuss later. At that time, with no literature or research available to suggest how feasible or effective a patients' library might be, the doctors decided to provide one and carry out their own research. The Regional Health Authority gave a grant which paid for the initial cost of about 400 books. The grant also covered the cost of purpose-built shelving in the main surgery waiting room and – a librarian's salary. A collection of audio and video tapes was added later. I was employed on a part-time basis to set up and run the library and do research.

The practice: setting and 'style'

Site The Dib Lane Surgery is definitely an urban practice, though not actually in the inner city. It has a fairly compact catchment area on one side of which is a pleasant leafy area of suburban housing; on the other, the edge of a large council housing estate. Most patients live locally, and cover a fairly wide cross-section of society.

Size The original two doctors (with about 5,000 patients) now have a third partner Dr Zelia Muncer. The list has increased to 5,700 and is growing. The GPs are supported by a medical team which has three practice nurses, a health visitor, district nurse and midwife.

The library as a resource

The books serve the whole practice team. One of the aims of the research was to see if the library would also be used by all the patients, not just middle-class or well-educated people. Would it reach people who did not normally buy books or go to local libraries? To find out exactly whom we were reaching and what they thought of the library, we gave each user a fairly detailed questionnaire. This asked (i) whether or not they found their book useful, informative or boring; and (ii) their social background and reading habits. The results were quite encouraging!

Almost all the readers claimed that they had learnt something useful from their books; very few felt the texts were too complicated or confusing. Middle class readers predominated, but others not in the habit of using the public library or reading regularly at home, also benefited. One striking feature was that women users outnumbered men by about 3:1. Even allowing for the fact that more women attend the surgery, this was a marked difference. Women readers also borrowed several times as many books as their male counterparts who usually took only one. The women – most of them aged between 20 and 40 years – tended to return and borrow several more.

Subjects of interest

The first selection of books was slightly haphazard, more or less one of everything found in the local bookshops. In 1980, much less information was directed at patients as compared to medical practitioners. We intentionally threw the net as wide as possible, including specifically medical subjects as well as books on welfare and social topics such as retirement, redundancy, caring for the elderly etc. Children's books were displayed to attract parents through their children. Indeed, the single most popular subject was child care, followed closely by fitness and diets – including books advocating a generally more healthy lifestyle.

The patients thus showed an encouraging interest in 'health' as opposed to 'illness'. However, books on particular illnesses were also popular, especially those describing chronic conditions such as arthritis, diabetes, back problems and migraine. Mental health – particularly anxiety and depression – was a favoured topic: cancer has only recently attracted much interest.

I personally believe that the library can help patients to gain a much better understanding of their condition and to feel more confident in helping themselves. Sixty audio cassettes were added to the library to assist patients who were poor or reluctant readers, but where books and tapes were both available, borrowers tended to prefer the books – except for tapes on relaxation. We acquired very good tapes on this topic from the 'Relaxation for Living Foundation'. Cassettes are a particularly suitable medium for teaching relaxation as you can actually relax while you listen. A book just cannot have the same impact. Commercial videos, although quite popular, are still exorbitantly expensive. Most of ours were produced by pharmaceutical companies.

Setting up a library

(i) *How much will it cost?* Cost depends on the size of the project. Our research grant bought a fairly comprehensive range of 400 books and purpose-built shelving etc. However, I have made up a sample list of 100 various titles which cost about £500. Covering to protect the books, and shelving would be extra.

(ii) *How much work?* The most time-consuming aspect is choosing and ordering the books and preparing them to go on the shelves. Once that is done, the reception staff could probably cover any necessary work in less than an hour a week, or a few minutes each day.

The books should be easily accessible, and available to patients whenever the surgery is open. Wheeling them out once a week or once a month is useless. It is important to have a system which enables patients to browse through the contents and find what they want without having to ask for help. That might be inconvenient or embarrassing. With the exception of tapes, all our stock is freely available on open shelving, where a very simple colour-coding system gives a guide to the subject matter: a coloured sticker on the back for child care, another for arthritis, diabetes, etc.

One of the niggling doubts about running a library is how to prevent the books from walking off! The borrowing system is kept fairly simple. Each book has a card inside the cover which contains the title and identification number. Borrowers simply fill in their name and address, hand it to the receptionist, and hopefully, return the volume after a statutory two weeks. A standard letter sent requesting the return of overdue books usually works like magic! Obviously, not always. However, there are no fines, as these could discourage or intimidate people nervous about using the library. Our overall stock loss has amounted to only about 5 per cent per annum. Another 5 per cent should be allowed for replacing books which are damaged or outdated.

Patient response

The library has been used consistently over the nine years, though numbers were rather inflated in the first year due to the novelty factor. On average, five or six items a week are borrowed, including tapes. But that greatly underestimates the actual use of the library. The number of people who browse through the books while they are waiting in the surgery cannot be estimated. People quite often ask for books on subjects which interest them and make suggestions about new acquisitions. The doctors and nurses can recommend books knowing the title is available.

Conclusion

Overall, the library has been a worthwhile project, but like all tools in health care, it has its limitations. Perhaps reading a book on giving up smoking is rather like reading a book on how to ride a bicycle – it is no substitute for actually doing it. But, considering factors such as the pressure of time on GP interviews, our experience has shown that a library can help patients understand their particular health needs better and also provide the motivation for them to adopt a healthier lifestyle which, after all, is the aim of the exercise.

Further information

Relaxation for Living Foundation, Dunesk, 29 Burwood Park Road, Walton-on-Thames, Surrey KT12 5LH. (Enquiries with self-addressed envelope please).

Address for contact

Clare Pace, Dib Lane Surgery, 112A Dib Lane, Leeds LS8 3AY.

12 Health Information

B Self-Help Health Information Services

ROBERT GANN, Director,
The Help for Health Trust, Winchester

SUMMARY

Public education, 'prevention' and personal responsibility feature in many major health-care proposals presented since 1980. The resultant growth in public interest and competence has spawned an amazing profusion of self-help literature, media coverage and community-based support groups. Ways in which a general practice library can help separate fact from fiction in written or recorded information have been described by Clare Pace. This paper outlined how a self-help information service, such as the one based in Southampton General Hospital, can complement and extend that function. The value of an easy, single-access comprehensive database which is available on subscription to people interested in setting up similar services, is discussed. Easy access to and reliability of information services must be assured.

Promoting mental health: Too much information?

People faced with threats to their health, independence and general wellbeing, are increasingly turning for advice and support to self-help and voluntary groups. Many types of self-help groups now operate in the UK – eg, The Spinal Injuries Association, The Mastectomy Association and The Hyperactive Children's Support Group. They offer information, practical help and mutual support to their members. There are at least 1,000 national self-help groups and many local groups so that in Wessex alone we have 2,000 groups.

Clare Pace has described the substantial literature and other printed materials and media programmes now available. Elliott Binns, in an article in the Journal of the Royal College of General Practitioners, also highlighted the increasing input from pharmacists and informal sources of information such as relatives and friends. Information is a valuable resource, but with so many wide ranging sources, where *can* people turn for *reliable* advice?

Information services

Information services have sprung up throughout the country, the most popular form being the telephone helpline. The first of these in Britain was 'Healthline', set up by the College of Health. Commercial organisations now sponsor many similar operations – some of which may offer truly remarkable opportunities. One, for example, advertised on the front page of a national paper, greets readers with 'So you are thinking of becoming a prostitute?'. Would calling a help-line and listening to a three-minute tape *really* help answer that question?

The Wessex Region Help for Health Centre

The Wessex Region Help for Health Information Centre opened at Southampton General Hospital in 1979, serving a largely rural population. Today the service has moved to its own premises in Winchester and provides the most comprehensive information about self-help groups and self-help publications available in the UK. The numerous leaflets on mental health are supplemented by popular medical books, many of which have been donated by the British Medical Association (BMA) in return for my having written 'What your Patients may be Reading' – a column which ran for two years in the 'British Medical Journal'.

The Centre receives many requests for advice on how to set up a self-help group; fund it; publicise it; and keep it going. Professionals, voluntary groups and individuals with a personal interest in such projects all use this facility.

Figure 12.1:

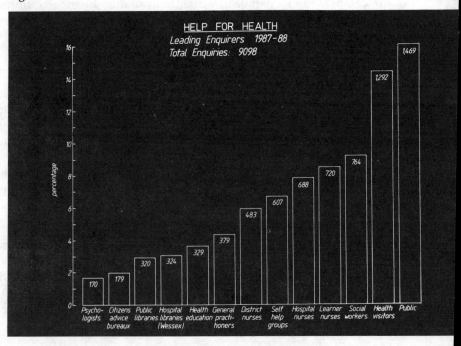

Phone-in service

The Centre's main activity is its phone-in service which puts people in touch with self-help groups anywhere in Britain. It provides a single point of contact, accessible to everyone. But people need services closer to their home town, and the Centre is encouraging GPs, health centres and health promotion departments to develop their own information resource.

Who uses the phone-in?

The service now receives over 10,000 enquiries a year. Figure 12.1 shows its users in 1987–8. The users today can be ranked in a similar way to that shown for 1987–8 in figure 12.1. Key professional contacts – health visitors, social workers, and GPs – are frequent users, and self-help groups also seek advice. The biggest change over the 10 years however, has been the increase in enquiries received direct from the public.

Three times more women than men are customers. This 3:1 ratio is constant for most health information services, both nationally and in the United States of America. This may well be because women seek information on behalf of their children and other members of their family (eg, elderly, dependant parents).

Coping with demand: self-help database

When Help-for-Health opened in 1979, it met with much suspicion and frank hostility – especially from hospital-based doctors opposed to the idea of patients having independent access to information about their own health. Now, the idea of self care is accepted and cartoons such as depicted by Figure 12.2 appear all the time.

Demands on the Centre grew so rapidly that in 1986, a database containing details of several thousand self-help groups, books and leaflets was set up to help the staff cope with the many and varied enquiries. This proved so effective, that the database (called Helpbox) is now provided on subscription to numerous other health authorities. Thus it (i) provides welcome income and (ii) enables people to set up similar centres without re-inventing the wheel (especially avoiding the time-consuming work required to gather the initial, reliable data).

On 1 April 1991, Help for Health became an independent charitable trust and moved to its own house in Winchester, providing a drop-in information centre, extra office space and meetings rooms.

Conclusion

The concept of self care is now well established. However, if 'ordinary' people are to become more confident about and competent in dealing with problems for themselves they must have ready access to reliable information and appropriate community resources. The Wessex Help for Health Centre and the general practice library in Leeds both go some way towards meeting those needs.

Figure 12.2:

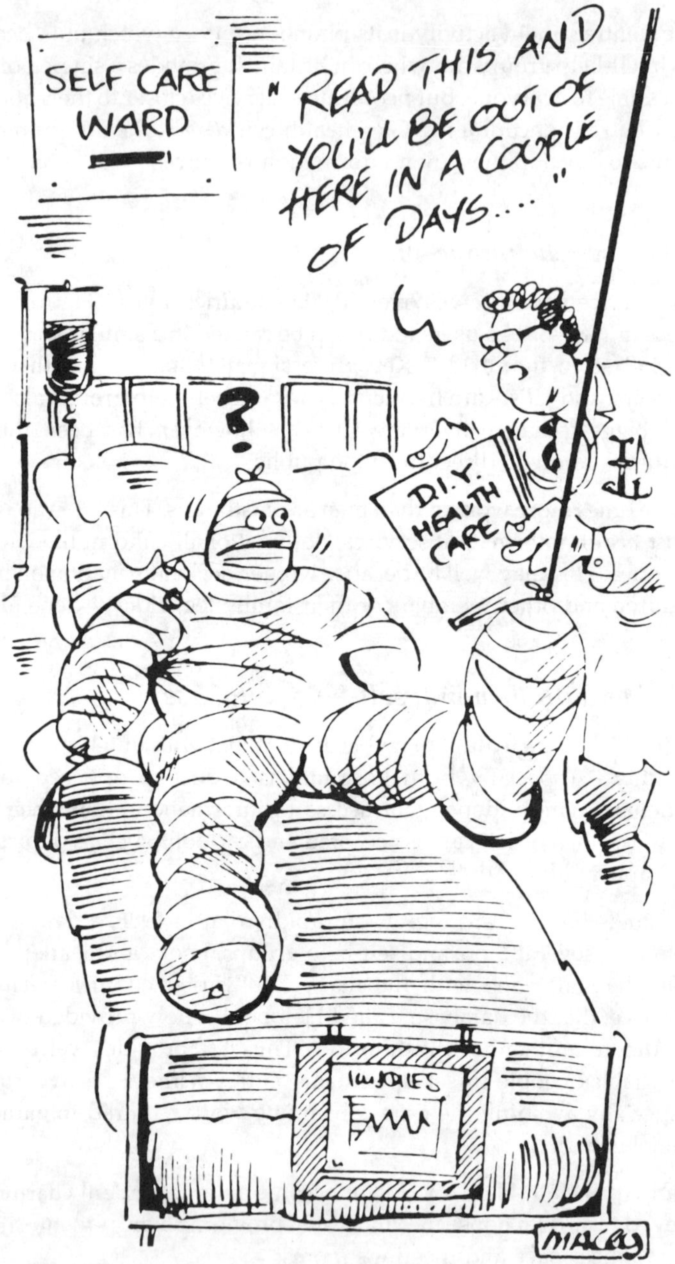

Kevin Macey/Health Service Journal

References

1. Elliott-Binns C P. Analysis of lay medicine. *J R Coll Gen Pract* 1986;**36**:542–544.

Further reading

Gann R. *The health care consumer guide*. London: Faber and Faber, 1991.

Address for contact:

Robert Gann, Director, The Help for Health Trust, Highcroft Cottage, Romsey Road, Winchester, SO22 5DH. Tel: 0962 849100. Fax 0962 849079.

13 Linking with Voluntary and Community Resources

A Home-Start Consultancy

MARGARET HARRISON, Director,
Home-Start Consultancy, Leicester

SUMMARY

Even the most delightful and most wanted infants can disrupt established (often cherished) adult routines, strain marital relationships and place heavy, consistent demands on parents. Many families with one or more pre-school children, run into difficulties. If not resolved, these can have serious effects on the immediate and long term wellbeing of both parents and children. HOME-START, a voluntary organisation, offers help to such families. Well-prepared, appropriately-matched and carefully-supported volunteers visit them in their own homes as often and for as long as necessary. Friendship, reliability and the opportunity to move from the client (receiving) to volunteer (giving) role are important aspects of the scheme.

'Hooray! Here comes Tuesday!'

HOME-START is a voluntary organisation which offers support, friendship and practical help to any family with at least one pre-school child when its members are experiencing stress and difficulties. Carefully-trained and 'matched' volunteers visit families in their own homes where their problems exist and their identity can be respected and protected. Visits continue for as long as is necessary; sometimes for a few months; sometimes for a few years. If it has taken years, or even generations for families to become overwhelmed by their many problems, it would be naive and insensitive to think solutions could be found in only a few weeks! My 17 years' experience working through HOME-START has proved that, with regular visiting over perhaps a two-year period, families with many problems often reach the stage where they can become HOME-START volunteers supporting others with problems similar to their own, with which they are now more able to cope. This is a very important aspect of the scheme.

The *volunteers* who support young families come from a wide variety of backgrounds – different ages, different education, different cultures. The *families* are referred mainly by health visitors (45 per cent of all referrals in 1989) and social workers; then – probation officers, teachers, home-helps, speech therapists and increasingly, as HOME-START becomes better known, families themselves. That is the very best form of referral. When families are referred, they are very often suffering from exhaustion and loneliness. They might be single parents, have low morale, over-high expectations of family life, over-high expectations of themselves as parents. Some parents have been brought up in care; others feel socially isolated. Many have a fear of failing; of not understanding. Like the mother who said she had been told to give her children more protein, but she was not quite sure what protein was, or where she should buy it.

HOME-START can turn apathy into energy; despair into hope. This is well demonstrated by the story of one little girl who named the family's volunteer, 'Tuesday'. Her mother, to quieten her frequent demands, used to say, 'Wait until Tuesday comes!'. Her happy response introduced this section.

Families and friends

Anna

Anna was a young mum, brought up in care herself. Her first baby, born when she was 15, died a cot death at the age of 11 weeks. Anna was quickly referred to us by the hospital medical social worker, when she was pregnant again. HOME-START introduced a motherly volunteer who got to know her, helped her to keep doctor and hospital appointments, and delivered urine samples for her. Anna and she planned for the baby together, but about four weeks before it was due, Anna suddenly rejected her volunteer. 'I don't want you coming here any more. You're bossy like all the rest. I've got a doctor. I've got a health visitor. I've got a midwife, a probation officer, a social worker. And I don't want you to come any more!' The volunteer replied, 'OK, that's your choice. I'm only a volunteer. You don't *have* to have me, although I must say, I really enjoy being with you.' Anna looked at her, and replied, 'Oh, all right then, if you want to, you can come.' That seems to have been the turning point in their relationship.

The volunteer's statement was very honest. HOME-START is a *voluntary organisation* and because we work through volunteers, *families do not have to* have us. Volunteers *choose* to be in the scheme, and the little phrase, 'the power of powerlessness', affects us very much. So many families want us *because* we have no authority. Anna had the baby; her volunteer was with her very regularly from when she took the baby home. In fact, a very close friendship developed and the volunteer was able to stay with Anna during the usual ups and downs of family life.

Jenny

Jenny was a single parent with three young children. She had recently been rehoused from a women's aide hostel, was on tranquillisers, and in an extremely nervous condition. When I first visited her as the HOME-START organiser, she talked non-stop about her 'nerves'. She attributed all her problems to her 'nerves'. I introduced a volunteer to her within a few days. We sat in her living-room, with two very pale little boys on the floor. They were just sitting. Just looking. With a frozen gaze – at nothing. There were no toys anywhere. Just Jenny, filling the air with her talk. The volunteer took a brown envelope out of the waste paper basket. Families like these so often get only brown envelopes don't they? She screwed it into a ball and rolled it along the floor to one little boy. He sat there – totally disinterested. She retrieved the ball and rolled it to his brother – without reaction. But she persevered, until one child rolled it back. Jenny stopped her torrent of words, laughed, and joined in. Probably the first time she had interacted positively with her sons for a long time. The ice was broken. I went back after the volunteer had been visiting for about six weeks. Jenny confided in me, 'We're more like sisters you know, me and Viv. We talk about anything and she comes when she says she will.'

Christine

Christine had two children – a three-year-old and a new baby. She was having sleepless nights with the baby, and also, regularly at 5.00 am, the three-year-old would get up, go into the kitchen, smash half-a-dozen eggs, tip the baby out of the cot, and generally wreak havoc. Christine was overwhelmed; her ordered routine and tidy home were threatened. Her response was to walk the streets, keeping the children out of her much-loved house. She regularly attended the local childminding group and the local play group, and was on anti-depressants. A HOME-START volunteer visited her regularly and within six weeks, Christine was off tablets and off the streets. 'What made such a rapid change in your life?' we asked. 'It was when the volunteer said "Contact me any time of the day or night; here is my phone number. If you really feel like throwing him out of the bedroom window, just phone me up and I'll come round right away". Christine never did need to phone the volunteer; just knowing that she could, took the pressure off.

HOME-START: Theory and practice

The late Mia Kellmer Pringle[1] said that children need love and security, praise and recognition, responsibility and new experience if they are to develop healthy minds and bodies. In HOME-START, very often, we first have to help parents experience these things themselves. They need praise and recognition. They need love and security. Maybe, just the knowledge that we will turn up when we say we will. They need to know they matter. They need new experiences and of course, responsibility.

Ann Dally, in her book *Mothers – Their Power and Their Influence*[2] says that children go through three stages of development:

(i) *Enclosure*, when children, up to the age of two years, need to be nurtured and are very dependent on the care-giver (usually a parent).
(ii) *Extension*, when the children are very much and increasingly influenced by other people; by the world at large. As children are extended by their parents they in turn extend their parents.
(iii) *Separation* begins with adolescence (12–14 years) and proceeds quite naturally to the point where, as young adults, children need their independence.

This model, I believe, explains much of the HOME-START approach. When families are referred to us they are at the enclosure stage. They need to be cherished and nurtured in their own homes where their problems exist. They need a time of dependency where they know another 'mum' will come and respond to what they need. The trick then, is to move them on to extension. There they can begin to seek and use other resources in the community – such as a drop-in-centre, a family centre or a health clinic. Other myriad services exist, but so often, at first, these families are not aware of their presence, or have insufficient confidence to contact or use them. Finally, we separate. They no longer need HOME-START. However, families very often return, perhaps a couple of years later, saying, 'I'm going through another bad patch. Can I have my volunteer back?' We are available for that.

Many families become volunteers. Ronald Laing said[3], 'If we take away people's deeds, like playthings from the hands of young children, they are bereft of their humanity.' People who have been on the receiving end of the welfare services, sometimes for quite a long time, often need to come out and volunteer. They gain enormous benefit from that experience.

HOME-START succeeds because it works very closely with statutory and voluntary agencies in the community through a management committee; through paid organisers and secretaries; through teams of volunteers who have been realistically recruited, carefully prepared, sensitively matched with only one or two families at a time, and then meticulously supported. The last is essential. Over 100 schemes operate throughout the UK and the average cost of HOME-START is £314 per year per family visited. In 1989, 15,000 children were supported in this way within their own homes.

Conclusion

Human problems require human solutions. Those which embrace qualities such as love and kindness, joy and understanding, respect, hope, and fun. So much can change just through having a friend; being alongside each other, genuinely caring and sharing and having fun together. Professional workers seeking ways to prevent the occurrence and effects of anxiety and depression should invest early in the care of families with young children who are experiencing stress and difficulties. HOME-START schemes offer a practical solution for many such young families.

References

1. Pringle M K. *The needs of children: a personal perspective prepared for the Department of Health and Social Security*. London: Hutchinson, 1974.

2. Dally A. *Mothers: their powers and their influence*. London: Weidenfeld & Nicolson, 1975.

3. Laing R D. *The politics of experience and the bird of paradise*. Harmondsworth: Penguin, 1967.

Further reading

Van der Eyken W. *Home-Start: a four year evaluation*. Leicester: Home-Start: Consultancy, 1982.

Address for contact:

Margaret Harrison, Director, HOME-START Consultancy, 2 Salisbury Road, Leicester LE1 7QR. Telephone: (0533) 554988. Fax: (0533) 549323.

13 Linking with Voluntary and Community Resources

B Camden Tranquilliser Services

RUBY TOVET, Project Co-ordinator,
Camden Tranquilliser Services, London

SUMMARY

Dependence on benzodiazapines is a well-recognised and widespread problem. *Camden Tranquilliser Services (CTS)* helps people who are having any difficulties with these drugs. Fully-recovered volunteer 'ex-users' and selected 'non-users', trained by them, run the services. Therapy consists largely of talking/listening and supplying long-term support via telephone contact, home visits, groups and one-to-one meetings. Clients are encouraged to stabilise, then reduce, the dose of benzodiazapines at their own pace, and are supported through the physical, emotional and mental adjustments which occur. The service (gently) helps people to face their pain, deal with it, and allow the change, which the organism is demanding, to take place. There is no alternative to this process if healing is to go ahead. Ex-user helpers need support themselves when the residual pain of their experience is re-contacted by doing this work. Client-response varies from one visit only, to staying with CTS indefinitely and working towards helping others. Ways are discussed in which GPs can help patients overcome their dependence and related problems (eg, by being non-censorious and patient), and coping skills which individuals may learn to use effectively (eg, relaxation, self assertion).

Background

Problems caused by long-term dependence on prescribed medication are well documented. *Camden Tranquilliser Services* were set up in North London in 1989 to help people overcome problems associated with dependence on minor tranquillisers – the benzodiazapines. I have worked as co-ordinator of the services since 1989. It is rare for people seeking our help to be taking only one medication. Some will also have been on, or still are on, major tranquillisers and/or antidepressant drugs. They are advised immediately, that the service can help them only with their dependence on benzodiazapines.

An ex-user of psychiatric services myself, I suffered the distress of long-term anxiety and depression in the 1960s and 1970s. I have no medical or pharmaceutical training, but for years have, as a qualified teacher and counsellor, helped people begin the self-healing and self-development process necessary after becoming dependent on tranquillisers. My work has been helped by skills first derived from my training as a teacher and counsellor, from personal experience of mental illness, and finally, from contact with the people themselves who have visited our centre – especially those who have recovered from this dependency and survived intact.

Cure and personal change

Everything that lives grows, and if an organism's emotional needs are ignored, suppressed or inappropriately deferred, distress emerges in the form of anxiety and depression. My very painful personal journey, and these later contacts with fellow sufferers have taught me that, when anxiety and depression are severe and prolonged and no longer responsive to well-tried methods of relief, the sufferer must undergo personal change before improvement can occur and dependence be overcome. No other solution is possible; continuing to take consciousness-altering substances merely succeeds in delaying the time when fundamental change must take place.

The process of change is slow and painful. Consciousness-altering drugs might be needed by some people at specific stages in their difficulties. They certainly saved me from the straightjacket or padded cell. However, taken for years, tranquillisers compound difficulties. Reasons for the underlying turmoil remain unclear and unresolved. Anxiety and depression continue, even if muted, and further distance individuals from participation in everyday activities and interests. When medication ceases, the suppressed emotions surface, as clearly illustrated by two examples quoted from participants at the centre:

(i) 'I couldn't cry at my father's funeral. My sisters thought I was hard. But when I came off my pills I cried for him every day for a month.'
(ii) 'I went on these pills when I was 16. Now, at 35, I look at my husband and daughter, and I wonder how I ever got mixed up with them.'

Making the change

There is no way of avoiding the pain associated with the changes required to overcome dependence on benzodiazapines. People fighting dependence on these drugs need exceptional support from as many relatives, friends and associates as possible. Each one of us must realise that we can make a unique contribution to someone else's welfare. Supporters must *accept* the validity of the drug-dependent person's experience and pain (ie, show empathy). That and/or sympathy provides reassurance; evidence that others do care; do understand; and are willing to provide *support*. This trust allows users to accept help; to use this to gain greater control over their daily lives; to grow in confidence and become more self-assertive. Self-assertion in turn allows people to have more obvious influence on what happens to them in their daily activities. This success helps dispel the frustration which, previously translated into depression, had led to inertia, isolation, and loss of confidence.

At this stage, surprising hurdles might appear. For example, partnerships can be threatened as an entirely new person emerges; one who disrupts established patterns of behaviour, patterns which reflected how one partner (the non-user) needed the other (the user) to be. By dealing with these and related problems, the user is encouraged to progress further (*expand*) – from an egocentric focus, to one which enables him or her to offer help to others and widen their scope of interests and activities.

Staffing and experiences

People dependent on tranquillisers need much time and varied types of help. Counsellors should be easily accessible by phone, letter or consultation over long periods of time. Participants in the programme need to mix with others like themselves, who are struggling with similar problems, to prove they are not alone. People who have already overcome dependence often provide the first ray of hope to newcomers. 'You had a 16-year addiction but now you're completely recovered? That's wonderful! You've made my day!' Benzodiazapine-dependent people need long-term encouragement and help to set up new friendships and social support networks. These are very important, particularly when attendance at the Centre finishes.

Ex-user helpers: Volunteers who have overcome dependence on benzodiazapines (ex-users) are valuable members of the Camden Services team. They are recruited and trained especially for the job and provide an immediate bond, based on understanding and acceptance, with participants. This relationship is often difficult to establish with a professional person, however necessary medical and pharmaceutical advice might be.

Volunteers must have recovered completely from their dependence. Many who have suffered long-term addictions before putting the experience behind them, find it impossible to help in the rehabilitation of other sufferers; the experience proves to be too painful. They cannot cope with the re-awakened distress. I understand this. I too found it very difficult at first to move from the position of being an ex-addict to helping people overcome their dependence on benzodiazapines. The work puts one in touch with pain, but once this is faced, acknowledged, and borne again, it dissipates, leaving the individual much better able to function than when the pain was present at a subliminal level. I work very hard to persuade others to face this pain and dispel it once and for all.

Non-user helpers: As there are insufficient volunteers from the ex-users group, we also recruit non-user helpers. Such people are expected to have some experience in dealing with emotional distress, and sympathy for people dependent upon medication. They undergo a training programme with my ex-user volunteers to get vicarious experience of what it is like to be on these pills for a long time. Sometimes they staff the helpline.

Progress

By using these resources in this way I have run a support group for 1½ years and I am about to set up another. We see people on a one-to-one basis also. A helpline is being developed and a home-visit scheme. The latter is necessary because many people become agoraphobic after taking these pills for a long time and need help to overcome this added problem, by being visited at home. The growth of a friendship network is also being encouraged.

Client response

Some people come only once. When they discover that we have no magic formula, as instant as the pills themselves, they turn away. It is hard to face the fact that something you took to make you better will also take a very long time and much effort to dispense with.

Others gain the moral support they need after attending several sessions. By spilling out their anger and expressing their distress, they discover that they are not alone. They feel better and can go away to get on with their own lives.

Still others come regularly and for a long time. It is extremely gratifying to see them changing their lives and gradually gaining control. The changes are amazing to behold as their initiative blossoms and their self-esteem is heightened. When they first come they seem far away, indistinct characters who gently come forward into focus as they work with us.

GP response

I am in contact with GPs in the Camden area through referral, letter, and increasingly, by visiting group practices to describe our scheme. GPs can help us with our clients in two important ways:

(i) By not insisting on the sudden or speedy withdrawal of the drugs.
(ii) By not blaming clients for their lengthy dependence.

Someone who has had a lengthy dependence needs to have it pointed out to them that they might be taking these pills for life. They ought to think about stopping, but they need to take their own time over it. Sometimes they need to wait until they can find a support group or other help, or until influences in their daily lives settle down and they can make a small reduction in the number of tablets taken. I tell them 'Don't make a reduction until it's a real one, one that you're not going to go back on.' I meet many people who, before they came to us, have had many relapses and so have suffered much unnecessary extra distress. It is essential to encourage patients to come off tranquillisers at their own pace with a little reminder every now and again, if they slow down.

Most people feel very ashamed about taking the pills, but these were prescribed in the first place and the patients received renewal prescriptions. It is not like taking drugs or alcohol for pleasure. Censure from a professional person creates very understandable and negative barriers. Our service then has to work through those barriers before we can inspire people with the confidence to take the first step towards independence from the drugs. Feelings of resentment are hard to overcome. Blame from any source is destructive.

I start from the existential position, ie, how the client is, and work towards how the client wants to be. Success may be decided by the availability of support and the number of options available. If clients can learn to use various techniques like relaxation, self-assertion and stress management, they begin to have confidence in their own ability to manage themselves and their surroundings.

Conclusion

Dependence on tranquillisers is a source of much anxiety, depression and distress. Perhaps with the help of caring people, the demand for such substances which we take from outside ourselves and put in, will diminish as people discover that they have the resources inside themselves to deal with the external problems.

Further reading

'Stepping Out' by Shirley Trickett, BBC. 1988. Booklet produced to accompany BBC's TV Day Time Live. Broadcasting Support Services, PO Box 7, London W3 6XY.

Address for contact:

Ruby Tovet, Camden Tranquilliser Services, Barnes House, 9–15 Camden Road, London NW1 9LQ. 071–911–0815

13 Linking with Voluntary and Community Resources

C A GP's Perspective

KATY GARDNER, General Practitioner,
Liverpool

SUMMARY

A community-based drop-in centre was opened on 8 April 1991 in a multi-racial inner-city area of Liverpool. The centre, which employs local staff, aims to provide contact with, and counselling and support services for, emotionally-distressed people in this area, particularly those who have lost or who never had effective contact with conventional health services. The project will also provide in-service counselling training for staff; will monitor research and evaluation studies relevant to the centre's aims and activities; will involve clients in management of the centre; and will develop outreach links into the community. Ways in which this project is being developed are outlined.

Background

Toxteth, where I have practised as a GP since 1978, is an inner-city district of Liverpool. Street riots made it the centre of media attention in 1981. Those disturbances, thought to be caused by racism and chronic disadvantage have attracted money from various sources over subsequent years; money which has enabled health professionals, such as myself, and community-based workers to set up projects designed to tackle at least some of the problems underlying the original unrest.

Despite their dramatic form of expression, I do not believe Toxteth's problems are unique. A previous speaker has described the 'tide of human misery' which comes through the GP's door. Toxteth is no exception. In order to avoid becoming depressed and anxious about this, I spend only two-thirds of my work time in the surgery. This need to get out of the office, to seek causes of and ways to stem 'the tide' has both directly and indirectly led to my involvement in projects such as the Granby Community Mental Health Project.

The Granby Community Mental Health Project

Our practice is situated in Granby, an area of Toxteth with a large proportion of black and ethnic minority residents. Poverty is widespread and so too is unemployment. In one street close to our health centre, 80 per cent of the men aged 16–64 years have no jobs. Many generations have suffered institutionalised racism and in Liverpool, the proportion of jobs filled by black people is incredibly small. The community also has many ethnic groups – like the Somali community whose members are not widespread in the rest of the United Kingdom. Their problems have been compounded by a massive and continuing influx of refugees whose personal stories are horrendous. Many of their relatives are dead or are confined to refugee camps in Somalia. The inner-city area also attracts people with mental health problems; drifters dependent on alcohol or illicit drugs, who occupy 'bedsit' accommodation and increasingly, swell the number of homeless.

The Health and Race Project

In 1985, the Liverpool Race and Health Project was set up to look at the health needs of black people. One area they studied was mental health: women from the Liverpool Black Womens Group had already identified this as an area of need after visiting black people in mental hospitals. A depressing picture emerged.

Many of the black community were very distressed: emotionally upset and isolated. They had little or no contact with the health services, because these were staffed mainly by 'white professionals' with whom they had little in common. For example, young black men felt unable to tell their own GP – 'I feel depressed.' Such an admission was unacceptable to themselves and, not without reason, they often feared it would be equally unacceptable to their doctor. This situation has serious implications for well-meant redevelopment programmes suggested for local community improvement. Some of these young people, poorly educated, unemployed, and living in unsatisfactory accommodation, also used alcohol or illicit drugs to ease their distress and boost their confidence. Without the professional support needed to help them overcome this dependence and rebuild their self esteem, few would be able to accept or use offers of jobs, training, or commercial initiatives designed to boost employment.

In 1987, the Health and Race Project attempted to determine how many of the patients in the mental hospitals in Merseyside were black. This study met with resistance from hospital psychiatrists. Many of them felt that the result of such a survey would be difficult to interpret, as no official data show what proportion of the UK population is black. However, the Project persevered, and a headcount showed that, in contrast to many similar studies in other parts of the country, the black population in Liverpool was under-represented among patients admitted to the local mental hospitals. Further examination of these results, coupled with information gathered by our own health centre, revealed that black patients admitted from our practice stayed for shorter (very short) periods and when discharged, were more quickly lost to follow-up than were their white counterparts. Reasons for this difference were unclear, but it seemed very likely that a black person admitted to an essentially 'white' institution might feel, or be made to feel, out of place and would become more distressed rather than comforted by the experience. When this disquiet was conveyed to the GPs, we supported early discharge – only to lose sight of the patient soon after. With such poor treatment, it was inevitable that the emotional problems would erupt again and precipitate re-admission, often under a Section of the Mental Health Act.

The Granby 'Drop-In' Centre emerges

In an attempt to address these problems, a drop-in day centre was proposed which would be open to people regardless of race, age, or sex. This multi-racial mix posed no problem in the Liverpool 8 area, although the same could not be said for some nearby districts with predominantly white residents.

The centre would seek to provide readily-accessible and acceptable premises; caring and supportive counselling services; and links between the black community and institutions responsible for mental health care in the statutory and voluntary sectors. It would aim to make and maintain contact with people who had lost or who needed contact with health services. Four major aims influenced the planning:

(i) *Training*: The Centre planned to recruit workers who lived in the area and to complement this local knowledge and inherent understanding with counselling skills developed via an in-service training programme. Counselling would be a main service offered by the centre.

(ii) *Research and evaluation*: It would be essential to determine what role the centre should develop in the community. Perhaps many of the people whom the project wished to contact would be too disturbed, or for various reasons, very reluctant to visit the centre. The project would need to define the size and nature of these groups, as well as monitor and evaluate the day-to-day activities and services offered. One of the facilities which could help bring more people to the centre and integrate it into the community would be outreach services.

(iii) *Community links*: Links with the community were already strong, because many of the people involved in setting up the project live locally. Some are professionals and most of them are black. They include social workers and a community psychiatric nurse. It was not so easy to appoint a psychiatrist. When the Granby project first started, psychiatrists were reluctant to be involved, because the scheme involved non-professional workers acting outside a hospital or clinical setting. This resistance has lessened, perhaps in part because of the growing acceptance of self-help models in health care. Such models interpreted literally, could be a cause for concern: they suggest isolation more than independence. But when the 'self' includes community support and community services, they provide quite an exciting innovation.

(iv) *Management* of the project would involve the clients themselves within the management structure – innovative and difficult though that step might be. A solicitor experienced in such matters was employed to work out a strategy for the formation and operational structure of a management committee.

Interim accommodation and action

Before the capital funds granted for the project were received from Urban Aid, or a suitable building was found, a drop-in service was run from our health centre. Most people who visited us were already in contact with the health services; three or four who had nowhere else to go and who were feeling miserable and isolated, enjoyed calling in for a cup of tea and chat once a week. But we did not reach the main client group for whom the project was designed. This was not surprising as a health centre is not the ideal place for a service of this kind.

Some girlfriends and wives, who are often kept awake until 5.00 am discussing their partners' problems, visit me in the surgery. Not surprisingly, women are often more stressed than men, since they must care for babies, homes and partners. I also see women whose male partners physically abuse them because they take their frustrations and anger out on the people closest to them. That is not new, but we all know how badly such behaviour affects individuals and families. As a GP, I hope that such men will be among those who come to the centre and benefit from that contact. I am however, willing to find that they do not want to go anywhere; that the centre does not meet their needs. But whatever the outcome, the Granby Community Mental Health Project is an exciting experiment. It is very important for me and my partners in the health centre to work closely with the community. We will provide an 'on-call' advice cover and will co-operate with the psychiatrist now working with the group.

Future plans

Funding for the first four years has been provided by Urban Programme development money. At the end of that time the project must find alternative sources of income. I am convinced that this project is a step forward and that bright ideas should not be stifled because of money worries. We need to listen to the voice of the community and to people other than professionals. For community health services to work effectively, participants must learn to listen as well as to speak, and to decide on action which represents composite, rather than merely an individual, official, or other narrow view.

Conclusion

Many people living in the community, who are emotionally disturbed have either lost, or have not had, contact with conventional health services. This problem is of particular concern in inner-city and socially-deprived areas. Means by which community-based services can reach these people, are urgently needed. A racially-mixed drop-in centre staffed by local workers encourages closer contact. Time will be needed to gain the trust and the confidence of the client group and careful evaluation will be necessary to determine both the effects of the initial services offered and how these might be developed.

Acknowledgements

Thanks are due to Dr Protasia Torkington from the Granby Community Mental Health Group for her help in preparing this paper.

Further information

Granby Community Health Group, Mary Seacole House, 91 Upper Parliament Street, Liverpool 8.

Address for contact

Dr Katy Gardner, Princes Park Health Centre, Bentley Road, Liverpool L8 3TX.

14 Mental Health Promotion in General Practice

CARYLE STEEN, General Practitioner,
London

SUMMARY

Mental health problems make up an increasing part of the workload borne by general practitioners and members of the primary health care team. The GP is well placed and increasingly well equipped to address these problems, and where appropriate, to practice preventive medicine and promote mental health. Ways in which this might be done in general practice include the use of multidisciplinary teams linked to and supported by other agencies such as community mental health and social services, and community-based voluntary and self-help groups. By working closely together, these services can provide comprehensive care appropriate for and readily accessible to the community they serve. Ways in which this type of practice has been developed in a London suburb are described, and the need for proper evaluation of the effects of this type of practice are noted.

Background

When I see vocational trainees in general practice dealing confidently and competently with mental health problems, I feel slight pangs of envy. In the 1960s, my generation of GPs had to learn slowly, rather at the expense of our patients. The only light in our darkness was Michael Balint who so wisely taught us to value our own emotional response to patients; to use that understanding; and also, to use ourselves as the drug[1].

The medical profession has learnt much about predisposing causes and management of mental illness in the intervening 30 years. Perhaps most exciting however, has been the growing interest and competence in prevention; in the search for ways to detect and ameliorate – even eliminate – much of the personal distress and economic hardship which mental health causes to patients, their families and on the wider stage, the national economy and health services.

GPs and health promotion

GPs are in an excellent position to practice preventive medicine and promote good physical and mental health. They have the marked advantage of being able to get to know many of their patients, indeed whole families, very well. They share the joys and sadness of major life events, sometimes meeting people for the first time as the result of unexpected crisis. GPs thus have closer and longer contact with their patients than any other professional group. This special relationship may be used to advantage when considering the promotion of mental health.

Many of the well-accepted causes of mental illness – personal constitution, childhood experiences, the vicissitudes of life, and socio-cultural factors – are no strangers to family doctors. Patients often present as a result of strains caused by poor housing, unemployment and poverty – conditions over which they and the GP might feel they have no control. However, a GP who is aware that these influences exist, will be alert to danger signals put out by his patients. For instance, Mrs Blogg's 'fluttery feelings in the stomach' and anxious expression, perhaps associated with her husband's redundancy, might well be the first signs of recurrent depression. The GP, aware of the patient's past history and current social difficulties, will be better able to diagnose the underlying cause of the presenting symptoms and treat them quickly and effectively.

I personally regret the reduction in home visiting. A very brief visit can provide a sharp snapshot of a person's life-style and circumstances. An out-of-hours visit to a young family, or a Sunday afternoon call to grandma, can reveal more about the family dynamics than hours of family therapy!

Despite the progress made in the diagnosis and management of mental ill health, some GPs still find it a difficult subject. Professor Goldberg has outlined the process of collusion (see Chapter 4). I would suggest that four main reasons underlie GP resistance to anticipatory care in this area:

1. *Tradition:* the medical profession has a long tradition of responding only to problems which patients present to them; of reacting to, rather than taking the initiative with, problems offered. A reactive stance might be justified in some cases of mental ill-health, because a problem perceived by only the 'professional' half of the doctor/patient relationship requires a very sensitive doctor indeed to help the patient also accept that problem. Insensitive interviews raise unnecessary hostility and delay clinical recovery. A skilled GP will create the climate necessary to gain the patient's trust and confidence.

2. *Job Satisfaction:* When heavy workloads put time at a premium, it is very satisfying to complete a task quickly and with good result. Physical illnesses seem to offer such opportunities more readily than do their mental health counterparts. The GP can follow a more precise process of investigation, continuing through a clearly-defined diagnostic procedure which combines clinical acumen with scientific (laboratory) investigations and provides a solution to the problem. The process is satisfying for both the doctor and the patient. Mental illness seems to be less straightforward; more prolonged. Results of preventive action in particular remain uncertain, perhaps for many years. But we should remember that this is true also for the prevention of physical ill health (eg, coronary heart disease).

3. *Time:* The diagnosis, prevention and management of mental ill health 'all takes a long time'. The same patients come back again and again. They often

make little progress if treated within the constraints of a 10-minute appointment schedule and can, by their frequent visits, put a strain on the system. However, a GP who recognises that an underlying problem is the probable cause of the presenting symptoms and needs skilled attention, will ensure that such patients are referred to appropriate sources of help. The time spent solving the problem need not be doctor time (see also Chapter 8).

4. *Pandora's Box:* Doctors who feel uneasy about dealing with mental health problems are often reluctant to disturb the status quo. They feel they might not be able to handle the contents of a Pandora's box once opened. Such fears should be allayed by learning new interview and management skills as outlined by Linda Gask (see Chapter 5). Indeed, many anxious patients need little more than the opportunity to share their concern with a doctor who is prepared just to listen.

I will now try to illustrate how, in our general practice, the primary health care team tackles these problems.

The James Wigg Practice

The practice is situated in a North-West suburb of London whose population of 13,000 is of mixed age, social class and ethnic origin. The practice operates from a health centre owned by the district health authority and we share the building with several tenants – currently the community mental health service, psychiatric nurses and midwives, RELATE (formerly Marriage Guidance) and the organisers of various classes for ethnic minorities and patient groups.

We *GPs are supported* by a staff of receptionists, practice nurses, attached district nurses, and health visitors who have specific responsibilities for the elderly and for young families. We have forged important links with the community psychiatric nurses, midwives and the Social Services. As part of this latter co-operation, a social worker spend two days each week in the practice. This service began 15 years ago, and the current incumbent, a fully-trained analyst, offers supportive/crisis psychotherapy and runs patient groups – in addition to providing advice on more traditional social work problems.

The psychiatric service provided by the practice has benefited greatly from a link set up 23 years ago with the Tavistock Clinic, our NHS facility for psychotherapy. A consultant psychiatrist, then interested in community health, placed members of his team in each of six local general practices. Clinical psychologists, therapists, senior registrars and the consultants took part. Each 'consultant', who stayed about 18 months in the practice, ran a weekly clinic and attended a weekly lunchtime staff meeting, where specific problems about referred patients or clinical topics were discussed. We found that this meeting provided much-appreciated support for the specialist who also gave a rich educational input to the practice[2].

Twelve years later we negotiated a similar agreement to obtain a child psychotherapist. The first consultant spent two years attending our baby clinics, helping mothers cope with very young babies and thus avert later problems. Her successor, a very senior child analyst, has helped us with older children. Half the patients described in her recent book on child sleeping problems came from our practice[3].

We also keep close contact with our local authority psychiatric department. The community psychiatric nurses have specialised interests and run fortnightly clinics for alcohol and drug-dependent patients in the centre – thus providing another valuable resource which is readily accessible to both patients and staff.

A *'health desk'* staffed by health visitors, and situated in the reception area, allows ready access to clients seeking information about medical or social matters.

Voluntary organisations are also welcome to meet us informally and discuss problems of mutual interest.

Multidisciplinary work can greatly help the patient, and we believe that working in this way has reduced our need to refer people outside the practice. However, the workers have to recognise their own roles and limitations when sharing care, and must be able and willing to support each other.

Linking preventive practice to life events

Rachel Jenkins alluded to the importance of recognising the natural sequence of life events common to us all and how this provides crucial periods in our development (see Chapter 2). An effective way of promoting mental health is to link action to key periods in this sequence.

Preconception

GPs have an excellent opportunity to counsel young women (and whenever possible, their partners) who actively seek advice about starting a family. Facts about the importance of diet, alcohol intake and smoking can be exchanged in return for information about the patient's present and past physical and mental health, personal relationships, and social situation – including support networks. Brief consideration of the impact a baby would have on this overall picture may prove enlightening. More opportunistic counselling should also be considered when women first come for contraceptive advice. Careful questioning can uncover plans, perhaps not fully realised by the woman herself, that she might have a baby 'shortly' – the contraceptive being used to control the timing of, rather than preventing, that event. A GP's intervention at this time, can be very influential, particularly for two high-risk groups – the deprived young girl who speaks impulsively about becoming pregnant, and the older career woman who plans to have a baby later in life.

Antenatal Care

Many GPs share antenatal care with hospital teams. We run weekly clinics with our midwives and meet after each session to discuss problems found on the day. As Debbie Sharp has shown (see Chapter 10B) women under extra strain and at risk of depression can often be identified during this time.

Measures can then be taken to provide the support needed and so avert the illness.

The health visitors and the midwives get to know each woman well. They run antenatal classes which include information about how to cope with *20 years of being a parent* – not just 20 hours of labour! The health visitors emphasise how to survive with small babies, and an evening meeting is held to involve fathers. They are a rather neglected group, often difficult to involve.

Postnatal care

Postnatal care has certainly landed in the GPs' laps. Young mothers bounce out of hospital so quickly! This can be a frightening prospect and experience for a first-time mother (and father) unless adequate support is provided to help with the inevitable demands of round-the-clock feeding, interrupted sleep and adjustment in former partnerships.

The health visitors keep regular contact with these families and run a postnatal support group. As a result of this continuing care – we see 99 per cent of our pregnant women – most of our new mothers attend postnatal examinations. These visits allows us to assess their mental health much more effectively than is usually possible at routine hospital follow-up appointments.

Baby clinics

Baby clinics run by the health visitors, with GPs in attendance, provide continuity of care for both mothers and infants. Indeed, I tend to call them *'ill mother'* rather than *'well baby'* clinics because mothers are often very worried about their baby's care. The reason for this concern might not be obvious and our child psychoanalyst has helped us solve many of the more difficult problems. For example:

We recently found that several babies attending the clinic were not putting on weight. There was no clear medical reason for this, but we found that their mothers were all preoccupied with what they should and could feed them. Questioning revealed that they had all been excessively upset by widespread media accounts about the dangers of listerellosis, 'mad cow disease' and salmonella infection. We GPs were unable to assuage their fears or persuade them to give the babies more food. The consultant however, helped us discover the underlying cause common to all these mothers – namely, their own early eating problems. Once this issue was addressed and discussed, the babies received adequate nourishment.

Children

GPs rarely see children unless they are brought by their parents because they are physically ill or because there are problems in the family. In our practice, school teachers often refer children, many of whom present with behavioural problems such as truanting, non-achieving and psychosomatic symptoms. We frequently take part in case conferences which discuss these children and their families. We also willingly get involved with family therapy and quite often call in Dad, visit everyone at home, or even talk over the problem with grandma. We make dual visits with the health visitor, and domiciliary visits with the family therapists employed by the district health authority, whenever this is thought necessary. In this way, we try to contain the problems and their management to resources available within the health centre.

Adolescents

Adolescents are a difficult group. They tend to see the GP as an authoritarian figure; someone out of touch with modern values and lifestyles and someone not to be trusted. An ability to dispel this image will give the GP an invaluable opportunity to raise some of the important issues relevant to the mental health of the emerging adult. Some GPs have taken the step to invite all youngsters on the practice list, when they turn 16, to attend for an informal discussion and explanation of their new rights as a young adult and to establish a personal relationship between the young person and the GP[4].

Working-age Adults

Difficulties with personal relationships – especially marital, family and work – are the reasons why many working-age patients visit their GP. Work is a very common source of stress and one worth investigating. Divorce is the all-too-frequent result of long-term pressures on marital and family partnerships. Our social worker, who has a particular interest in relationship-based problems, has helped many men and women resolve these difficulties by holding individual and group therapy sessions.

Unwanted pregnancies are far too common. With so many effective means of contraception available, we need to examine why so many women fail to use them either at all, or without effect.

Pre-retirement counselling is an important service offered by some of our GPs who have attended special courses. There is a high percentage of *successful suicides among men* in this age group. For many, their work has become equated with personal esteem and independence. Retirement can also highlight marital problems which have remained unresolved for many years.

Alcohol dependence presents frequently and in many guises. Once 'unmasked' the problem is discussed and we refer those patients who decide they really want to change, to the community psychiatric nurses who run regular clinics in the centre.

The elderly

The new NHS contract requires GPs to contact their over-75 clients annually. In practice, most GPs know this group well, and with the help of health advisers to the elderly try to meet their needs. We find isolation and depression are common syndromes needing intervention.

Chronic illness patients and carers:

GPs are generally much better at caring for the ill than they are at looking after the family and carers of patients who have a severe or prolonged illness. For example, our psychotic patients are well-supported by the CPNs and our practice nurses. The latter monitor the card index we keep for patients on depot injections and notify the GPs if any are overdue. Our district nurses, aided by the health visitor, provide care for the chronically sick and elderly patients.

However, illness can cause a great deal of distress to the family as a whole as well as individual members. This distress can also affect carers outside the family. The GP, being aware of the difficulties, can help carers by referring them to local self-help groups and other relevant, often voluntary organisations, who supply on-going support. I have been most impressed by the skills developed by these groups. Their *management of bereavement* is a good example of how the mutual support provided by the group can lessen the need for formal bereavement counselling, a service which we provide to help prevent post-bereavement depression.

Conclusion

GPs, by the special nature of their personal and often prolonged contact with people of all ages in their practice, are well-situated and increasingly well-trained to diagnose and manage mental illness. Most important, they can use their position and skills to prevent or lessen the adverse effects of such illness and promote sound mental health. They do this best when working as a member of a multidisciplinary team whose combined skills can provide easy access to a variety of services. These may be complemented by links with other government agencies, voluntary and self-help groups. The prevention programme may be enhanced by following a life-event sequence, beginning with pre-conception counselling and continuing stepwise, to care of the elderly and bereavement. Careful evaluation of this type of practice is needed to prove that it does indeed *prevent* the development of mental illness. How this might be done poses a challenge to the many individuals and organisations involved.

References

1. Balint M. *The doctor, the patient and the illness*. London: Pitman Medical, 1957: 2nd ed 1964: reprinted 1968.
2. Brook A, Tempeley J. Contribution of psychotherapists to general practice. *J R Coll Gen Pract* 1976;**26**:86–94.
3. Daws D. *Through the night: helping parents with sleepless infants*. London: Free Association Books, 1989.
4. Donovan C F. Is there a place for adolescent screening in general practice? *Health Trends* 1988;**2**;64.

Address for contact:

Caryle Steen, The James Wigg Practice, Kentish Town Health Centre, 2 Bartholomew Road, London NW5 2AJ.